D1094589

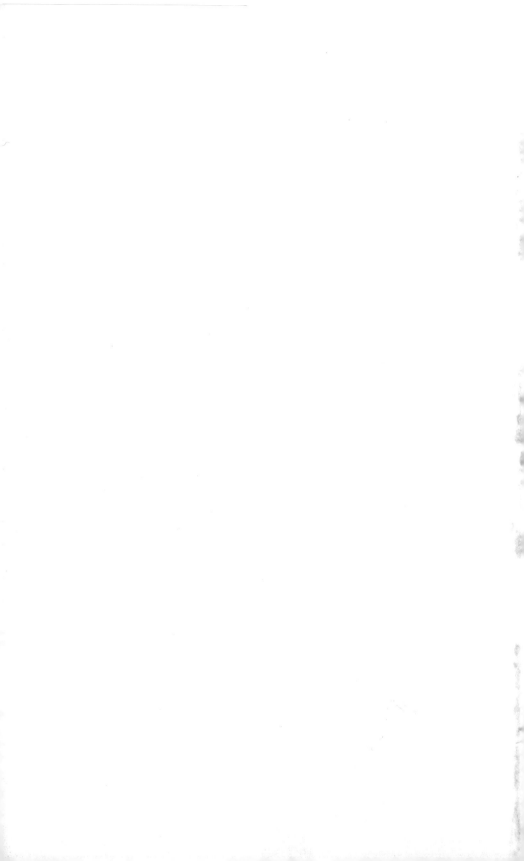

THE VETERINARY CLINICS OF NORTH AMERICA

SMALL ANIMAL PRACTICE

VOLUME 16 / NUMBER 5
SEPTEMBER 1986

DENTISTRY

Patricia Frost, D.V.M., *Guest Editor*

W. B. SAUNDERS COMPANY
Philadelphia   London   Toronto   Mexico City
Rio de Janeiro   Sydney   Tokyo   Hong Kong

W. B. SAUNDERS COMPANY: West Washington Square
                          Philadelphia, PA   19105

The *Veterinary Clinics of North America: Small Animal Practice* is covered in *Current Contents, Science Citation Index, ASCA,* and *Index Veterinarians.*

The *Veterinary Clinics of North America: Small Animal Practice* is also published in Japanese by Gakusosha Company, Ltd., Tokyo, Japan, and in Italian by Antonio Delfino Editore, Rome, Italy.

THE VETERINARY CLINICS OF NORTH AMERICA   ISSN 0195-5616
September 1986   Volume 16—Number 5

The Veterinary Clinics of North America is published six times each year by W. B. Saunders Company, West Washington Square, Philadelphia, Pennsylvania 19105, at Hampton Road, Cherry Hill, New Jersey 08034. Second class postage paid at Cherry Hill, New Jersey 08034. Subscription price is $60.00 per year. There is a postage charge of $7.50 for subscriptions billed to U.S. addresses and shipped outside the U.S. POSTMASTER: Send address changes to W. B. Saunders Company, West Washington Square, Philadelphia, Pa. 19105.
   The editor of this publication is Diane Ramanauskas, W. B. Saunders Company, West Washington Square, Philadelphia, Pennsylvania 19105.

   Printed by the Maple-Vail Book Manufacturing Group, York, Pennsylvania.

Contributors

GARY BEARD, D.V.M., Goodwood Animal Hospital, Baton Rouge, Louisiana

BEN COLMERY, III, D.V.M., Westarbor Animal Hospital, Ann Arbor, Michigan

PETER EMILY, D.D.S., Director and Chief of Animal Dentistry, Colorado State University College of Veterinary Medicine and Biomedical Sciences, Fort Collins, Colorado

DAVID ARTHUR FAGAN, D.D.S., Director, The Colyer Institute, San Diego, California

PATRICIA FROST, D.V.M., Veterinary Dental Service, Roosevelt Roads Naval Station, Ceiba, Puerto Rico

GARY S. GOLDSTEIN, D.V.M., Veterinary Dental Clinics, Houston, Texas

COLIN E. HARVEY, B.V.Sc., M.R.C.V.S., Diplomate, American College of Veterinary Surgeons; Professor of Surgery, Department of Clinical Studies, University of Pennsylvania School of Veterinary Medicine, Philadelphia, Pennsylvania

B. JEAN HAWKINS, M.S., D.V.M., Orchard Animal Clinic, Boise, Idaho

DONALD L. ROSS, D.V.M., M.S., Veterinary Dental Clinics, Houston, Texas

CHARLES A. WILLIAMS, D.V.M., Director, Blue Cross Animal Hospital, Fairfax, Virginia

Contents

of orthodontics such as how teeth move, length of treatment, and limits to movements, and equipment and materials are considered in this article.

Some of the clinical problems most frequently seen in
veterinary dentistry and their surgical solutions are discussed. Extraction of teeth, surgical repositioning of teeth,
tooth transplant, oral abscesses of tooth origin, impaction
of teeth, repair of maxillary canine oronasal fistula, and
simple techniques for oral wiring are among the issues
considered.

The author describes the techniques and complications of
maxillectomy and mandibulectomy and summarizes results
of these procedures from several series of cases.

The author discusses the elements necessary for establishing a successful veterinary dental practice.

FUTURE ISSUES

November 1986
> VIRAL DISEASES
> Richard B. Ford, D.V.M., M.S., *Guest Editor*

January 1986
> ZOONOTIC DISEASES
> John R. August, B.Vet. Med., M.S., M.R.C.V.S., and
> Andrew S. Loar, D.V.M., *Guest Editor*

March 1987
> NON-CARDIAC SURGICAL DISEASES OF THE THORAX
> Dennis D. Caywood, D.V.M., M.S., *Guest Editor*

PREVIOUS ISSUES

July 1986
> COMPUTERS IN VETERINARY PRACTICE
> Brian R. Smith, M.B.A., P.E., *Guest Editor*

May 1986
> REPRODUCTION AND PERIPARTURIENT CARE
> Cheri A. Johnson, D.V.M., M.S., *Guest Editor*

March 1986
> CANINE UROLITHIASIS II
> Carl A. Osborne, D.V.M., Ph.D., *Guest Editor*

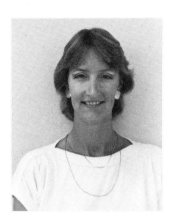

Foreword

Veterinary dentistry is a field in veterinary medicine that has been growing in leaps and bounds during the last 5 years. There are two new veterinary dentistry texts out, an active American Veterinary Dental Society, and numerous continuing education seminars for practitioners. This issue of *Veterinary Clinics of North America* is designed to be an additional source of information for the students, practitioners, and clinicians who are interested in the field of dentistry. It includes an article on the approach to diagnosis and treatment of dental disease, whether you are dealing with a domestic cat or dog or an exotic animal such as an African lion or a crocodile. In depth, up-to-date articles on the separate areas of periodontics, endodontics, orthodontics, restorative dentistry, and oral surgery are presented. An article on feline dental disease will bring the veterinarian up to date on dental problems seen in the pet cat. Finally, an article about setting up your own veterinary dental practice will provide valuable information for those veterinarians interested in expanding their practice into the dental field.

I would like to thank the authors for the time and effort put into their contributions. They are veterinarians and dentists whose expertise comes from extensive experience with veterinary dentistry. Many are private practitioners who were the founding members of the American Veterinary Dental Society and are active lecturers at continuing education programs on veterinary dentistry around the country.

I would also like to thank W.B. Saunders Company and Diane Ramanauskas for the opportunity to serve as Guest Editor for this issue. It was a project I was fortunate to have the time to take on during my stay in Puerto Rico, while my husband completes his commitment to the Army Veterinary Medical Corps.

PATRICIA FROST, D.V.M.,
Guest Editor

Box 3404
Roosevelt Roads Naval Station
F.P.O. Miami, Florida 34051

0195–5616/86 $0.00 + .20

Diagnosis and Treatment Planning

David Arthur Fagan, D.D.S.*

Most individuals subscribe to the notion that dental disease is an exclusively human frailty. However, a close look at the relevant veterinary literature will reveal that animals are afflicted with the majority of the dental and maxillofacial diseases and disorders seen in humans. This includes, but is not limited to, the following items: chronic sinusitis, severe genetic malocclusion, dental caries (tooth decay), destructive periodontitis (both local and generalized of all varieties), debilitating facial trauma, massive periapical abscessation, chronic draining oral fistulas, and a variety of facial and oral cancers. The patient population seems to include the entire spectrum, from aardvark to zebra and an assortment of avian and reptilian species, as well as both large and small domestic species. Altogether, an indication of too much disease to go unrecognized or remain untreated.

If veterinary dentistry is to continue to grow as a recognized clinical modality, its practitioners must develop the clinical prowess to recognize oral disease before it becomes terminally destructive. Veterinarians are faced with a learning situation similar to that faced a number of years ago by dentists, when the legal profession laid the clinical responsibility for the early detection of oral cancer directly upon the shoulders of the dental profession via the doctrine of "respondiat superior," or vicarious liability.

In a clinical environment, the responsibility for the timely detection of both dental and oral diseases rests with the veterinarians and their para-professional staff of animal health technicians and assistants. Most veterinarians, I believe, are genuinely sincere in their desire to accept this clinical responsibility. Obviously, however, this implies an adequate comprehension of the workings of the vertebrate mastigatory apparatus, as well as an understanding of its

*Director, The Colyer Institute, San Diego, California

most common failings. The assertion that "They didn't teach me anything about dentistry in vet school" does not absolve one of clinical responsibility.

The following material represents an attempt to summarize what is required to adequately diagnose and treat the most common veterinary dental disorders. It is generally well accepted that the understanding of any disease complex is completely dependent upon a thorough understanding of the normal state of affairs. All practitioners must have a fairly comprehensive grasp of the range of variations customarily seen in the healthy individual. This is particularly true when the patients in question embody such an extremely wide range of sizes, shapes, and functional variations as those seen in the animal kingdom.

FACTORS RELATED TO INFORMATION GATHERING

The essential ingredient for effectiveness in any clinical endeavor includes both an accurate comprehension of what is to be accomplished, as well as an understanding of the primary motive for accepting the clinical responsibility to do so. The way to acquire begins with a thorough understanding of what the clinician is expected to examine, including an exact definition, if possible, and ends with a familiar outline of the steps necessary to accurately realize the expected objective in an efficient and orderly manner.

GENERAL APPRAISAL OF THE EXAMINATION SITE

The predominant feature of many mouths is quite often the teeth. A tooth is a small, bone-like structure, usually found attached to or imbedded in the jaws of animals, that is used to masticate its food. Teeth serve a number of important functions for their owners, including the following: prehension of food, deglutition (in some fishes and snakes), incising of foodstuffs into bite-sized pieces, crushing of food to begin digestion through insalivation, acting as weapons for protection and to secure food, functioning as primary tools (the beaver, for example), acting as a sexual attraction, and assisting in reproductive behavior.

The original architectural form of the primitive tooth-like projection, or denticle, is that of a solitary cone. Embryologically, all denticles originate from ectoderm and are therefore characterized as specialized dermal structures like hair and fingernails. Teeth are composed of a combination of three dental tissues—*enamel*, the white, compact, and very hard calcium crystaline rods that cover and protect the crown of the tooth; *dentin,* the chief substance or tissue of teeth that consists of a solid organic substratum, infiltrated with lime salts, and permeated by numerous branching tubules that contain processes of the connective tissue cells that line the tooth's pulp chamber; and *cementum,* the thin layer of bony tissue covering the root of the tooth that differs from ordinary bone in that it contains a greater number of Sharpey's fibers.

All teeth can be divided into three functional parts—a *crown,* or portion protruding into the mouth above the soft tissue of the jaw and covered with enamel; a *root,* or portion covered with cementum that is used to attach the tooth to the jaw bone; and a *neck,* the portion located between crown and root.

By modification in response to functional demands over the years, teeth have evolved into four basic structurally functional forms. The *incisor* is a wedge-shaped form with a long, conical root used to cut objects. The *canine* is an enlongated conical form that is used to puncture, hold, or tear objects. The *premolar* is a transitional form with a crown usually composed of two or three small cones fused together usually with one or more long roots. The *molar* is a broad, squarish form designed to grind or crush objects and with a crown composed of multiple small cones called cusps.

The teeth encountered by a veterinary dental clinician represent as many variations and extraordinary forms as there are different species. The alligator has a very simple cone-shaped tooth, whereas the leopard seal has a row of premolars shaped like Poseidon's three-pronged scepter with beautifully sculptured miniature flame-shaped enamel cusps.

INVERTEBRATE DENTITION

Not all members of the invertebrate class have teeth, but when teeth are present, they are *analogous* to the teeth of vertebrates because they are usually oral organs that perform the same function as the denticles of vertebrates; they are not *homologous* with the teeth of vertebrates, however, because they may not have the same tissue of origin or similar structure (for example, the claw of a crab). The dentition of invertebrates varies in number from none to one (the beak of the cuttle fish or the claw of the lobster) to over 40,000 in the mouth of the snail.

VERTEBRATE DENTITION

With vertebrates, however, true teeth are the rule, not the exception, and are mostly confined to the oral cavity in the bones

and cartilage of the head and face or even the esophagus in some of
the snakes. Vertebrate denticles come in an enormous variety of
sizes, shapes, and quantities per mouthful. They vary in number
from none in the anteater, to 1 in the norwhal, to 6 in the elephant,
to 32 in man and the old world monkeys, to more than 100 in some
cetaceans. But regardless of their quantity, they can all still be
characterized as one of the four functional forms noted above; that
is even true with respect to the denticle or beak characteristic of
avian species. The eagle may only have one hooked "tooth" attached
to its stiff upper lip, but it still functions as the entry mechanism to
the digestive system.

HOW TEETH ARE ATTACHED

The teeth of vertebrates are all attached by one of four basic
methods. A *fibrous membrane* does the job for sharks and rays. An
elastic hinge works for most fishes, although some fishes and reptiles
utilize the method of *ankylosis*, or the continuous ossification between teeth and jaw bone with no intervening membrane. The
ankylosis method is divided into three styles depending upon how
the tooth relates structurally to the surrounding bone (that is, on a
pedestal, to the side of the jaw—usually lateral, or in a socket).

The fourth method of attachment is common to all mammals
and some reptiles; it involves the use of an intervening ligamentous
structure called the *periodontal ligament*. This ligament is embedded
into the cementum layer of the tooth on the one end and extends to
anchor the tooth to the surface of the surrounding specialized bone,
called the alveolar process, on the other end. The unique feature of
this method of attachment is that the alveolar bone is invaginated to
intimately surround the entire root(s) of the tooth, to form a bony
socket or crypt that is architecturally very sound. This type of tooth
attachment with its modified form of periosteum is called a gom-
phosis. It is a very sophisticated suspension apparatus which has
more in common with a wrist or ankle joint than with the other
types of tooth attachments mentioned above. Again, there are three
subcategories which relate to crown-to-root ratio. Of interest is the
fact that the continuously growing incisor tooth of rodents is one of
these subcategories with the ligamentous attachment.

The ligament represents a very effective method of absorbing
and distributing the forces of mastication without undue injury to
the surrounding bone. It is because of the unique relationship
between the periodontal ligament and the surrounding bone that
mammalian teeth can be so easily repositioned or relocated within
the jaw by the light forces utilized in the practice of orthodontics.

Sudden, sharp or excessive forces to the tooth can, and in fact do occasionally, injure the ligament, much like a similar force would injure or "sprain" an ankle joint. The muscles of mastication in humans are capable of closing the mouth with about 250 to 300 pounds per square inch of biting force. When this load is "dropped" suddenly onto a cusp-tip of a tooth, say 1/100th of a square inch in cross section, it is not at all unlikely to realize a local force on the order of magnitude of 25,000 to 30,000 pounds—certainly enough to injure the ligament or fracture a tooth. In the larger or stronger carnivores, needless to say, the load is proportionally greater.

THE MASTIGATORY APPARATUS

The manner in which all these teeth, in all these different species, come together is referred to as their method of articulation or interdigitation, or occlusion. It is this articulation that enables all these individual denticles to operate as a single functional apparatus that structurally occupies the upper end of the digestive system. Clearly this apparatus comes in a wide variety of sizes and shapes designed to do an infinite variety of chores for its owner. For the veterinary dental clinician, however, some generalization is in order to reduce the matter to a manageable mouthful. It may prove helpful to think of the mastigatory apparatus as if it were a *picket fence*, in which case its owner inherits only three things:

1. The size, shape, and number of pickets or teeth (the dental formula: 0 to 40,000).

2. The length and shape of the fence or jaw bone (the arch-form: curved in a Boxer Dog versus long and thin in the Caiman).

3. The way the fences fit together (the temporomandibular joint, and the occlusion [aardvark versus crocodile]).

It is a bit more complicated than this, of course. What is not relevant here is the multitude of details available from numerous texts on comparative anatomy and osteology. What is of significance here is a practical method that will enable the clinician to rapidly and dependably correlate appropriate treatment alternatives with known anatomic variations, in order to facilitate the implementation of an effective treatment plan to correct the patient's problem.

The mastigatory apparatus in all vertebrates functions as a result of the balanced interplay between three independent, but related, biological entities:

1. The teeth, or the complete set of pickets along the fence.

2. The temporomandibular joint, or the hinge that facilitates the articulation of the fences.

3. The major muscles of mastication, or the movers of the fence

along the hinge axis during articulation, which, in mammals, include the following:

- a. Masseter—Short stroke/high power.
- b. Internal pterygoid—Short stroke/high power.
- c. External pterygoid—Moves the articular disc.
- d. Temporalis—Long stroke/medium power.
- e. Buccinator—Holds bolus of food on the occlusal table of teeth.

A TOOTH IDENTIFICATION SYSTEM

As a result of the influence of dental insurance carriers, most dentists treating humans utilize a system of nomenclature known as the "universal tooth numbering system" to identify teeth. This system assigns each of the human's permanent teeth a number from "1" to "32" and each of the 20 primary teeth a letter from "a" to "t." This system works quite nicely for humans because the majority of people have 32 teeth. However, the diverse nature of the veterinary dental patient population requires a more versatile system of nomenclature.

PALMER'S METHOD

The Palmer Notation System was developed before the dental insurance companys' system and has been used by some dentists for many years. It easily meets all veterinary dental requirements. The system is quite versatile, easy to use and understand, and precisely identifies a tooth by virtue of its location and function.

Individual teeth are identified according to the following three factors:

1. The function of the tooth (i = incisor, c = canine, p = premolar, m = molar).

2. Its location in relation to the patient's midline.

3. The quadrant of the mouth in which it is located (upper versus lower and right versus left).

Imagine that you are looking at the mouth of the patient through the cross hairs of a telescope, which divides the mouth vertically along the midline or midsagittal suture line and horizontally along the patient's plane of occlusion. Then the four quadrants of the dental arch (sometimes incorrectly referred to as an arcade, which is in fact an arched, covered passageway) are referenced with a small 90 degree angle:

upper left . . . . | _____ and upper right . . . .   _____ |

lower left . . . . | and lower right . . . . |

When the vertical line is to the *left* of the tooth number ($\lfloor$ 3), the designation represents a tooth or the quadrant on the left side of the patient. When the vertical line is to the *right* side of the tooth number (3 $\rfloor$), the designation represents a quadrant on the right side of the patient's mouth.

Tooth numbers *above* the horizontal line refer to maxillary, or upper arch teeth, whereas tooth numbers *below* the horizontal line represent mandibular, or lower arch teeth. Putting it all together, then, the upper right third incisor is designated in this way: i 3 $\rfloor$. The designation m $\overline{1}$ represents the lower left first molar. This nomenclature system can be applied to any species with any number of teeth. Moreover, the system is quite similar to the method generally used by veterinarians and other scientists to express the dental formula for a particular species. For example, the following is the permanent dentition "dental formula" for humans and the Great Apes:

$$ i \; \frac{2 \mid 2}{2 \mid 2}, \; c \; \frac{1 \mid 1}{1 \mid 1}, \; p \frac{2 \mid 2}{2 \mid 2}, \; m \frac{3 \mid 3}{3 \mid 3} = 32 $$

This is the formula for the rat:

$$ i \; \frac{1 \mid 1}{1 \mid 1}, \; m \frac{3 \mid 3}{3 \mid 3} = 16 $$

DEFINITION OF THE TASK

The basis of modern clinical therapy is diagnosis, which presupposes that disease can first be accurately identified and then effectively eliminated by the application of the appropriate treatment. The procedure by which the information required to make a valid diagnosis is obtained is directly related to the success of the treatment plan, because the diagnosis itself is based upon an assumption of valid observation and accuracy of information. It is not possible to overemphasize the importance of an efficient, disciplined procedure for collecting the material necessary to make a valid diagnosis. The apparent ease with which some clinicians arrive at a final diagnosis does not necessarily represent a tendency toward snap judgment. Rather, astute diagnostic prowess reflects the experienced clinician's ability to reduce large quantities of historical and factual data to a relevant minimum, while at the same time surveying the entire scope of inquiry and field of examination in a swift, but orderly, manner.

It is not the intent here to provide a shopping list of possible diseases with highlights of their cardinal signs and symptoms. The objective of this article is to present a summary of background information as well as a procedural outline to encourage the systematic collection of available information upon which a diagnosis is based by illustrating some of the diversity, similiarity, and common denominators present in the customary veterinary dental patient population. Information about equipment and instrumentation necessary to provide treatment is provided elsewhere and is readily available. The issue at this point is to understand, as accurately as possible, the range and scope of the field of investigation.

Veterinary dentistry can be defined as that branch of the veterinary healing arts that relates to the oral cavity and its associated tissues, including the teeth, and that is concerned with the diagnosis and treatment of its diseases, as well as the restoration of defective and missing tissues. Five general categories of clinical veterinary dental care can be identified, and they are characterized by the clinician's *motive* for undertaking that type of clinical task.

Preventive dentistry is concerned with the maintenance of the mastigatory apparatus and its associated structures in their normal functional state, including the prevention of all adverse systemic disease or disorders secondary to an oral problem.

Operative dentistry is concerned with instrumental procedures by which the integrity of the teeth is restored or repaired, thereby maintaining the efficiency of the individual's entire mastigatory mechanism and preventing deterioration of the patient's general health. This includes all oral surgery.

Prosthetic dentistry is concerned with the design and fabrication of all artificial appliances intended to replace missing parts of the oral cavity and/or face including, but not limited to, the teeth.

Cosmetic dentistry is concerned with the repair and restoration of decayed, broken, and/or defective teeth primarily to improve their appearance rather than their function.

Forensic dentistry is concerned with matters of public debate suitable for a court of law, including disease or body identification, and any application of the principles of law and justice as they relate to the practice of veterinary dentistry.

If the examining clinician grasps the functional significance of the object being examined and is keenly aware of the particular motive that prompts and justifies undertaking the task of diagnosis, he or she must determine how best to proceed in order to produce a maximum of results with a minimum of time and stress.

THE EXAMINATION PROCEDURE

The complete visual examination remains a bit of a gray zone in dentistry. Most agree that the patient should have one, but it remains unclear how often the patient should have an examination, or what kind of examination it should have, or who should pay for it. Unfortunately, too few clinicians get around to really doing a thorough job, and fewer still legibly or completely record what they find or don't find. Consequently, the literature abounds with advice to "malpractice proof" your technique and your records. The most commonly recommended solution is to establish a standard examination routine, and **always** do the same routine, and **always** record **all** of the variations or abnormalities. In this way, if there are no notes on the patient's record, it can be assumed that there was no abnormality at that time. When the routine is habit, the result is thorough and the time to complete it is minimal.

The only way to truly comprehend the range and diversity of accepted variations in clinical normalcy is to actually examine many, many individuals in an orderly and systematic fashion. Obviously, once the clinician is familiar with the basic anatomy of the head and neck, the signs and symptoms of oral disease become more apparent.

The best time to begin the evaluation of the oral problem of a particular patient is the first time you see that patient. There is no other time you can truly obtain that all-important first impression. Later on, the clinician will come to see exactly the same things that everyone else sees. It is appropriate during the first visit or sighting to make tentative decisions that can be confirmed or discounted later upon closer examination. Before the patient is approached too closely, restrained, confined, immobilized, or transferred to a shipping container, observe as much as possible in order to form your first impression, and then, as you approach the patient more closely, continue with the remaining items of your routine and complete the examination.

Following a complete general survey of the patient's past health record and with the first-impression factors foremost in mind, the examiner should undertake a detailed and systematic examination of the entire mastigatory apparatus. The procedure begins with the head and neck, proceeds to the face and lips, and then enters the oral cavity, traversing the buccal mucosa and contiguous structures to the hard and soft palates, the tonsillar region, the floor of the mouth, the tongue, the gingivae, and finally the teeth. The examination should be carried out systematically and routinely in this or a similar manner so that no portion will be overlooked.

The procedure recommended here is based on the concept that the examiner has learned how to examine the oral cavity, knows what to expect in the normal patient, and is aware of what variations of the normal should be considered potentially pathologic or abnormal.

If diagnosis is to be complete and dependable, and if obscure lesions are to be noted with any regularity, the technique of oral examination must be careful and exacting and should include more than just a "check-up" of the teeth. The oral cavity, like the eyes, represents a "window" to the patient's general internal well-being. Numerous systemic disorders manifest themselves with early, subtle signs or symptoms in and about the oral cavity.

An examination procedure that considers all of the essentials is as follows:

THE HEAD AND NECK

1. From a short distance away, study the patient's face for facial symmetry of hair, lips, whiskers, and facial moisture. See if the patient holds its head in a peculiar fashion.

2. Watch the patient walk and move about in order to notice unusual or atypical movements of the head, which is a sure sign of disorder.

3. Look at the eyes for discharge, droopy eyelids, photophobia, and protruding or bulging eyes. Look the patient in the eye for signs of alertness, depression, uneasiness, fear, apparent pain, and so on.

4. With the patient secured with a minimum of physical restraint or chemical sedation, palpate and percuss the sinus areas, looking for inordinate tenderness or actual response to pain.

5. Run your fingers over the bony portion of the head, face, and jaws, searching for bony asymmetry, irregularity, hemiatrophy, hemihypertrophy, or soft-tissue lesions, tumors, or discharges. Is there infection, neoplasia, or muscular enlargement?

6. Feel the motion of and within the temporomandibular joint, looking for crepitus, obstruction, tenderness, clicking, or snapping sounds.

7. Palpate the thyroid region of the trachea for the thyroid gland, outlining the gland for size and degree of firmness, and then run your fingers down the surrounding region of the neck, looking for enlarged cervical lymph nodes.

The Lips and Breath

1. Using the length of the thumb against the opposite fingers and occasionally their tips, beginning in the upper right corner of the mouth and proceeding around the lips to the upper left and then lower left and finally lower right, palpate all of the lips for evidence of cracking, fissuring, ulceration, or swelling of the soft tissues, salivary glands and ducts, and muscles of the area. Missing teeth, anatomic peculiarities, and incorrect positioning of the teeth will perpetuate a variety of mucocutaneous lesions. Inspect the physiologic and anatomic features of the lips in both health and disease for form, position, function, color, and texture. Look at the skin around the lips for ectodermal dysplasia, color uniformity, and condition of the hair, coat, and whiskers. Feeling through the cheek, palpate along the biting plane of the teeth (plane of occlusion) for irregularities in the alignment, which is a good quick indication of the ability to effectively masticate food. Finally, examine the nostril inside and out for lumps, trauma, foreign bodies, discharge, and normal moisture. This shouldn't take longer than 30 seconds in the absence of abnormality.

2. Pull the lips forward and invert them with the fingertips. Inspect the labial and buccal mucosa for color, texture, glands, ductal orifices, and attachments of the frenula. Look and feel for foreign bodies, sialoliths, or fibrous nodules. With a fingertip, compress the attached gingiva in an obviously healthy region and note the capillary refill rate.

3. With the lips retracted, smell the breath. Under ordinary circumstances, the breath of a patient with a normal healthy mouth does not attract the attention of the examiner. Good oral health has no odor. Disagreeable odors may be found in association with poor oral hygiene related to dietary lack of abrasivity, periodontal disease, rhinitis, sinusitis, necrotizing gingivitis, bronchiectasis, lung abscesses, and gastrointestinal upset. As a general rule, any oral, gastric, or respiratory disease or disorder may result in an obviously noticeable oral aroma.

4. Look at the alignment and articulation of the dentition, particularly the midline at the central incisors for symmetry, evidence of trauma, and/or malocclusions.

Inside of Mouth

1. Prop the mouth open. Use a discarded 1 cc syringe casing that can be quickly trimmed to the desired length with a standard toenail-trimming instrument and placed between opposing canine

teeth or premolars. Twist a length of quarter-inch adhesive tape around the middle to act as a "rip-cord" in case it needs to be retrieved suddenly. This type of mouth prop is not only radiolucent, but provides an excellent anchor to which to tie off the endotracheal tube to eliminate undesirable irritation of the trachea from movement of the tube while working in the mouth. With the mouth open, note the overall "cleanliness factor" of the oral cavity or the lack of it. Notice the consistency of the saliva (thin, watery, ropy, thick, syrupy, discolored). Excessive saliva tends to obscure dental disease, so it is best to wipe off the excess before proceeding. Inspect the palate, rugae, oropharynx, tonsillar tissue, and throat for form, color, and function.

2. Grasp the tongue with a dry gauze sponge and examine it for symmetry and taste bud pattern, tumors, self-inflicted trauma or cuts, foreign bodies, and bruises, particularly the posterior lateral surfaces. **Do not pull** the tongue forcefully! It is relatively easy to injure its nerve supply or to tear one or more of the numerous delicate muscle attachments. Notice what a normal tongue looks like, particularly the underside.

3. Palpate the medial and lateral walls of the mandible for exostoses or signs of fracture, and then the floor of the mouth by pressing the finger of one hand into the palm of the other hand held under the chin. The thin oral mucosa under the tongue will adhere to the dry skin of your fingers or to a dry gauze, so be careful not to tear the mucosa during this procedure.

THE DENTITION

Finally, look at the teeth. Gently hold the tongue out of the way, examine the teeth for proper and expected tooth form, alignment, enamel covering, level of gingival epithelial attachment, depth of gingival crevice, alteration of gingival coloration, mobility of teeth, discolored teeth, carious lesions (decayed teeth), periodontal disease, abrasions, or unusual functional contours of the teeth.

Note the difference between actual dental formula and expected dental formula (missing and/or supernumerary teeth are much more common than most clinicians expect). Feel the teeth with the fingertips for sharp points, fractures, split or loose teeth, irregularities in the plane of occlusion, and overall functional analysis of the masticatory apparatus.

The instruments and materials required to accomplish all of the above are minimal and need include only a small reflective mouth mirror, a sharp explorer or small needle held at the tip of a hemostat, a periodontal probe to measure gingival pocket depth, and a few dry gauze sponges. Of course, good illumination is a primary prerequisite for any examination. The patient should be positioned comfortably for ease of access to all areas of the mouth.

Keep in mind that this is an examination of the *entry mechanism* to the digestive and respiratory systems, not simply a look-see at the biological box where the teeth are stored. There are a number of good texts available (see references) that provide additional details on the subject of oral diagnosis.

Generally, carnivores are easier to examine than herbivores because they are able to open their mouths wider. The examination of herbivores usually requires a greater dependency upon deftness of finger. But it is possible to develop the sense of touch to the point that a great deal of the foregoing, except discoloration, can be recognized by "braille."

RADIOGRAPHS

Radiographs, when correlated with the case history and clinical examination, represent a most important supplemental diagnostic aid. There are numerous pathologic entities that cannot be detected by any other method and many other diseases, like cysts, tumors, and neoplasms, that only an accurate radiograph will reveal while they are still incipient. For these and other reasons, a radiographic series should be routinely taken whenever the opportunity provides itself or if disease is discovered or suspected. Detailed radiographic procedures are described by a number of authors (see references). Regardless of the technique used, however, any good radiographic series should include a sharp image of the anatomic region desired, with minimal distortion and proper contrast between tissues of differing densities and sufficient normal area surrounding the pathologic region to provide adequate comparison. A good-quality radiographic series is a tremendously valuable supplemental diagnostic aid, and its radiographic interpretation is invaluable.

Unfortunately, not only do poor-quality radiographs yield very little in the way of dependable information, but they quite often provide misinformation. If you plan to take x-rays, complete the series accurately, interpret the results completely, and make notes in the patients records that can be understood 5 years later. Obviously, a fundamental prerequisite for interpretation is an understanding of what constitutes normal and adequate illumination.

SUMMARY

It must be emphasized that any examination of a supposedly healthy patient must be thorough and careful, for the early detection of disease demands that minute and inconspicuous deviations from the normal be evaluated carefully. The detection of disease occurs during the examination procedure, and from a practical point of view, it appears that clinicians employ at least the following three types of examination, depending upon circumstances: (1) the comprehensive examination; (2) the screening examination; and (3) the emergency or limited examination. Although the latter two types represent a justifiable compromise with respect to the comprehensive examination in light of limitations of time or resources, the general inaccessibility of the patient in veterinary practice suggests that one should make the most of the opportunity for examination when it presents itself. A complete, thorough examination is not, by definition, a time-consuming and expensive procedure, particularly if there is no disease present. Exam-related expense is more a function of a differential diagnostic effort once clinical abnormality is detected, and then it is certainly justified.

The term "diagnosis" originates from a Greek word meaning to distinguish or to discern. For the clinician, it refers to the process of identification of a disease by investigating, in all their manifestations, the signs and symptoms presented by the patient. The word diagnosis describes not just a "disease identified," but the *process* by which the identification is made. The procedure for making a diagnosis includes the following four primary steps:

1. Collection of the facts.

2. Analysis of the data for relative importance.

3. Correlation between synthesized data and descriptive features of suspected diseases.

4. Selection of the disease that best explains the collected facts and apparent disturbed physiologic processes of the patient.

The process of diagnosis usually results in the naming of a disease. It is well to remember that a name is only a shorthand method of describing a set of signs and symptoms characteristic of a particular disease state. Emphasis should always be focused upon the clinical facts collected, not on the name of the disease selected.

Oral disease in animals results from an extremely diverse variety of environmental, dietary, and genetic circumstances. The clinical appearances of the disease process can vary considerably within a single species and may vary enormously from one species to another, particularly considering the contrasts between some captive environments and other natural habitats. For a variety of reasons, oral disease represents one of the most thoroughly studied of human ailments, and from a radiographic perspective alone, presents more than 20 major diagnostic categories. In spite of all this potential for diversity, from a practical point of view, the vast majority of disorders associated with the mastigatory apparatus of animals may be described as belonging to one of four basic groups, which tends to imply specific categories of treatment planning:

1. Developmental and congenital defects (includes dental caries).
2. Maxillofacial trauma.
3. Periodontal disease.
4. Trauma to the teeth.

The selection of a rational treatment plan for any disease is, of course, dependent upon the accuracy of the original diagnosis. Although dental treatments can be relatively complex, their successful implementation is simply a matter of preparation, combined with the availability of proper materials and access to the instruments and equipment necessary for their intended manipulation. Once a diagnosis is made, the treatment alternatives become rather limited and straightforward.

Today, the clinical practice of veterinary dentistry must concern itself with the rapidly growing discipline of disease prevention as well as changing trends in disease management theory. This changing scene suggests that early detection and prevention will play an important role in the future of all aspects of clinical practice.

REFERENCES

1. Colby, R. A., and Kerr, D. A.: Color Atlas of Oral Pathology. Philadelphia, J. B. Lippincott Co., 1971.
2. Collins, L. H., and Crane, M.: Internal Medicine in Dental Practice. Philadelphia, Lea & Febiger, 1965.
3. Colyer, J. F.: Dental Disease in Its Relation to General Medicine. London, Longhans, Green & Co., 1911.
4. Colyer, J. F.: Variation and Diseases of the Teeth of Animals. London, John Bale, 1936.
5. Ellis, R. G.: The Classification and Treatment of Injuries to the Teeth of Children. Chicago, Year Book Publishers, 1960.
6. Fagan, D. A.: The pathogenesis of dental disease in carnivores. In Proceedings of the American Association of Zoo Veterinarians, 1980.
7. Goldman, H. M. (ed.): Periodontal Therapy. St. Louis, C. V. Mosby Co., 1964.
8. Kerr, D. A., Ash, M. M., and Millard, H. D.: Oral Diagnosis. St. Louis, C. V. Mosby Co., 1959.
9. Page, R. C., and Schroeder, H. E.: Periodontitis in Man and Other Animals. New York, S. Karger, 1982.
10. Nizel, A. E.: Nutrition in Preventive Dentistry: Science and Practice. Philadelphia, W. B. Saunders Co., 1972.
11. Schnebitz, H., and Wilkins, H.: Atlas of Radiographic Anatomy of the Horse and Dog. P. Parey, 1968.
12. Stafne, E. C.: Oral Roentgenographic Diagnosis. Philadelphia, W. B. Saunders Co., 1963.
13. Sorrin, S.: Habit: An Etiological Factor of Periodontal Disease. Dental Digest, 41:291, 1935.
14. Tiecke, R. W., Stuteville, O. H., and Calanera, J. C.: Pathologic Physiology of Oral Disease. St. Louis, C. V. Mosby Co., 1959.
15. Zontine, W. J.: Canine dental radiology and radiographic development. J. Am. Vet. Radiol. Soc., 16(3):75–83, 1975.

The Colyer Institute
P.O. Box 26118
San Diego, California 92126

Dentistry   0195–5616/86 $0.00 + .20

Intraoral Radiology

*Peter Emily, D.D.S.**

Intraoral radiology, as the term states, is the placing of film (nonscreen type) into the mouth for radiography of a particular tooth, quadrant, or segment of mandible or maxilla. It has the advantage of clarity and definition of the subjects because of the absence of superimposed images of the opposite arch seen in extraoral radiography. Intraoral radiography is an excellent technique for mandibular and maxillary diagnosis when teeth are involved.

The disadvantages of the intraoral radiograph are the mouth size in the smaller breeds of dogs and cats and the restrictive confines of the mouth structures, such as the shallow dome of the palate, necessitating the bending or shaping of the film to accommodate these confines. This technique must take into account the shapes or bends placed into the film when positioning the x-ray tube for proper alignment.

The parallel and the bisecting angle techniques for proper intraoral radiography will be discussed, as will equipment, film type, technical values, and film processing.

This article will include a particular application of intraoral radiography: early diagnosis of missing teeth in dogs. This technique is useful when early diagnosis of missing teeth in dogs is necessary, as seen in our show dog clients with Doberman Pinschers and Rottweilers (four or more missing teeth is a disqualification in these breeds). Many other breed standards call for full dentition, with missing teeth being a serious fault. This is a financially rewarding procedure as well as a practice builder.

FILM TYPE

Intraoral film used in human dentistry is quite adaptable to veterinary use. The film itself has a firm but flexible polyester base.

*Director and Chief of Animal Dentistry, Colorado State University College of Veterinary Medicine and Biomedical Sciences, Fort Collins, Colorado

It adapts easily and is transported smoothly through the rollers in the new automatic processors. Also, this film base does not absorb water; therefore, it dries rapidly in the drying chamber. An emulsion of silver halide crystals mixed with gelatin is spread in an extremely thin layer over both sides of the base. Films for film holders and cassettes are packaged in a box, with each film individually wrapped in a black paper envelope. A film packet is made to be placed in the mouth; therefore, it has an outer wrapping of paper to protect the film from moisture and light. One side of the wrapping is stippled; this helps prevent slipping when the film is positioned in the mouth. This stippled side is *always* placed on the side facing the x-rays. Within the packet on the other side of the film is a lead foil backing, its purpose being to absorb as much exit radiation passing through the film as possible. It also helps to prevent fogging (darkening of the film) caused by secondary radiation created in the tissues behind the film. Immediately surrounding the film itself is a black paper envelope.[1]

Single film packets are used if only one copy of the x-ray is desired. A double film packet containing two separate films can be used if duplicate copies of the radiograph are needed.

The speed of the film denotes the rapidity with which the film becomes adequately exposed. Basically, the speeds are slow, medium, and fast or "high" speed. All other factors remaining constant, the slow-speed film requires the longest exposure time, whereas fast film requires the shortest time and therefore exposes the patient to the least amount of radiation.

There are two basic types of human intraoral films best suited for veterinary dentistry; each is named according to the radiographic technique with which it is used. With periapical film, which is used for small dogs and cats, as the name implies, the root apex of the tooth and the surrounding structures are of prime interest when this type of film is used in human dentistry. There are three sizes of periapical films. No. 0 is 7/8 by 1 3/8 inches, for use with the smallest dogs and cats. No. 1 is 15/16 by 1 9/16 inches, when a narrow film is recommended. No. 2, the standard size, is 1 1/4 by 1 5/8 inches and is designed for routine use. Occlusal film, for medium- to large-sized dogs is of ideal size. On this film, we can view a cross section of the teeth or a large section of palatal, mandibular, and maxillary structures. This technique is employed for determining the location of cystic lesions, impacted teeth, salivary duct stones, bone fractures, or for any instance in which the area of interest is larger than the area of the periapical size film. The occlusal film is 2 1/4 by 3 inches and it may be used intraorally or extraorally, depending on the situation.

EQUIPMENT

X-ray Units

A standard dental x-ray unit is recommended for optimum ease of use and for those practitioners who do extensive veterinary dentistry. The dental x-ray unit is small in comparison with other units. It can be stored against an operatory wall, taking up very little space and standing ready for immediate radiographic diagnosis. New dental x-ray machines vary in price from $2000 to $10,000, but there are many used dental x-ray units of the old type available from dental supply houses. These are x-ray units turned in for credit by dentists who are upgrading their office equipment. These units can be purchased for $100 to $500 and are very serviceable for veterinary use. In fact, they often produce x-rays of superior quality to the newer units owing to the lack of x-ray scatter controls.

Veterinary X-ray Units

Veterinary x-ray units are adequate and functional for oral radiography. The disadvantage is only in the ease of manipulation and range of movement.

Processing Tank

A portable developing tank (from Schein,* catalog #189-4677, $129.95) is recommended for speed, ease, and portability; however, standard developing equipment can be used as well. The use of dental x-ray hangers is necessary to hold the intraoral film for processing (Fig. 1).

PROCESSING A FILM

Before processing, all films must be identified in some manner to avoid confusing them with films of other patients. One method is to place the film packets in an envelope marked with the patient's name as soon as they are exposed. In the dark room, make a notation on the envelope of the number of the film rack on which the films have been placed. Upon completion of the drying time, the developed films are put back into the envelope until they are mounted or stored.

Film packets must be stripped of their outer protective wrapping. Remove the films from the packets, holding the edges of the

---

*Henry Schein, Inc., Port Washington, New York.

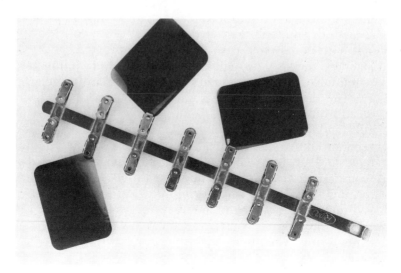

Figure 1. Dental x-ray film holder with multiple film clips.

film rather than the flat surfaces, and place them on a film rack to be developed and fixed.

A recent advancement in film processing is the automatic film processor. There are several different brands on the market, all of which function basically on the same principle. Once the film is stripped of its protective wrapping, it is inserted in a slot, picked up by revolving rollers, and carried through the respective tanks (developer, fixer, and so on). In a matter of 2 to 6 minutes, the film is emitted from the drying chamber ready for mounting. In another type of processor, the films are stationary in the unit and the respective solutions are dispensed separately by timing devices.

An option with most units is the daylight loader, a protective cloth with elastic cuffs that lets you strip the film and place it in the processor without being in a darkroom. This easily adapts to chairside processing, if this is preferred.

If there is a disadvantage to using these units, it would be that the radiograph might be slightly fogged because of the special high-speed chemicals used and the higher temperature of the solutions needed to speed up the processing time. This fogging, if present, is usually not that objectionable when weighed against the advantages.

FILM MOUNTING

The types of mounts and mounting procedures used are a matter of the veterinarian's preference. There is a mark on the film that is called the "dimple" or the "dot," depending upon which side of the film you are viewing. If the films are mounted so that they coincide with the teeth as you look at the patient's teeth, the dot side of the film should face you as you view the mounted x-rays. The alternate method would be viewing the films from the lingual side of the teeth; in this case, the dimple side of the film would be facing you (Fig. 2).

Reminders

1. The stippled white surface of the film always faces the x-ray tube when placing intraoral or extraoral film.

2. For films that are to be placed in a permanent record, do not "short cut" the processing steps. The exposed film must be developed, fixed, and washed exactly as directed.

3. When stripping the film, make sure your fingers are dry. Avoid fingerprinting the emulsion.

TECHNICAL VALUES FOR INTRAORAL FILM

Dental X-ray Unit

For small dogs and cats, 40 to 50 kVp and 8 to 10 MAS should be used. For medium to large dogs and cats, 50 to 65 kVp and 10 MAS should be used. Focal distance is 10 to 12 inches, exposure time is 1/10 to 2/10 seconds.

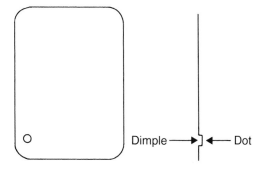

Figure 2. Front and side views of intraoral film.

Veterinary X-ray Unit

Exposure time and technique values used may vary depending upon the x-ray unit used; however, experimentation with your particular machine will soon show optimum values. The approximate values are 60 to 64 kVp and 100 MAS at 1/15 to 1/12 seconds with focal distance of 10 to 12 inches.

INTRAORAL TECHNIQUE

There are two basic intraoral radiographic techniques: the parallel and bisecting angle techniques.

THE PARALLEL TECHNIQUE

The parallel technique is one in which the long axis of the structures or teeth to be radiographed, the film, and the x-ray head or tube are parallel to each other (Fig. 3). This is a very accurate technique, but it is extremely difficult to obtain in intraoral radiography owing to the shape of the intraoral structures—that is, the shallow palate and short sublingual areas.

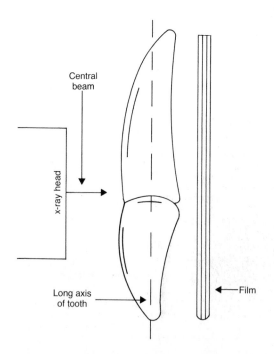

Figure 3. Parallel technique for intraoral radiography.

The parallel technique produces the most accurate images of the teeth because it follows more of the principles of accurate shadow casting. The conditions that must be fulfilled to cast a shadow of an object as accurately as possible as applied to radiographs of the teeth are: (1) the tooth must be parallel and as close to the film as possible, and (2) the source of the x-rays must be small and as far from the tooth as possible.

The two obvious differences between the parallel and the bisecting angle techniques are film placement and the distance from the target of the x-ray tube to the film (target-film distance).

The term parallel technique indicates the manner in which the film is placed (parallel to the long axis of the tooth in question). In order to do this, the film must be positioned at a greater distance from the tooth to escape the restrictions of the oral anatomy. The first condition for accurate shadow casting is therefore only partly fulfilled, and the film is in closer proximity to the tooth in the bisection of the angle technique.

The central x-ray is directed perpendicular to both the film and the teeth because they are parallel to one another. If you notice, after film placement, that a slight angle is formed by the teeth and film, a satisfactory shadow will be cast by directing the central x-ray perpendicular to the teeth. However, if the angle is greater than 15 degrees, you should direct the x-ray according to the bisecting angle technique. Failure to do so results in an elongated image. There will be dogs and cats in which it will be difficult or even impossible to come close to paralleling the film with the teeth because of the intraoral anatomy.

THE BISECTING ANGLE TECHNIQUE

This is the technique of choice, for it allows for the limited confines of the intraoral structures. Because of the irregularities in the make-up of the oral tissues, the film cannot always be placed parallel to the teeth being radiographed. When the teeth and the film are not parallel with one another, the x-ray may produce a shadow on the film that is either shorter or longer than the teeth themselves. To obtain a shadow equal in length to the teeth, the bisecting angle technique is used.

The success of this technique is based on the theory that if two triangles have a common side and two equal angles, they are equal triangles. Therefore, simply put, the central beam is directed per-pendicular to the line that bisects the angle formed by the film and long axis of the tooth (Fig. 4). The film can be placed or modified to accommodate the intraoral structures, and a clear image, neither

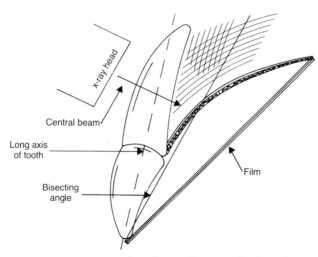

Figure 4. Bisecting angle technique for intraoral radiography.

elongated nor foreshortened, can be obtained. The central beam and tube head must be directed and placed at the correct lateral angle in relation to the head and muzzle to prevent superimposed structures and accurately produce images through the interproximal spaces when taking lateral views. These exact tube-head positions for all projections can be seen in the figures in the following section (see Fig. 10).

EARLY DIAGNOSIS OF MISSING TEETH

For this procedure, the occlusal, nonscreen type of dental film (Kodak, Df-50, ultra-speed) is used. Follow the manufacturer's instructions for the technical values and processing of this film. This is a technique to determine the presence, number, and type of unerupted permanent tooth buds in the mandible and maxilla in 9- to 12-week-old puppies. The exact principles of radiography are not necessary, for we wish only to see if tooth buds are present. If elongation or foreshortening occurs, or if the exact centering or location of the tooth buds in the film is malpositioned, it is not detrimental. We wish only to ascertain their presence or absence.

PROCEDURE

An approximation of the bisecting angle technique discussed previously will be used for the procedure. The puppies are tranquilized with a medicament of choice, such as acepromazine or

Text continued on page 815

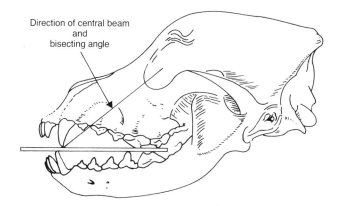

Direction of central beam
and
bisecting angle

Figure 5. Position of film and x-ray beam for an anterior radiograph using the bisecting angle technique.

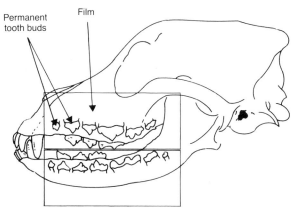

Permanent
tooth buds

Film

Figure 6. Lateral view of proper placement and area covered by x-ray film.

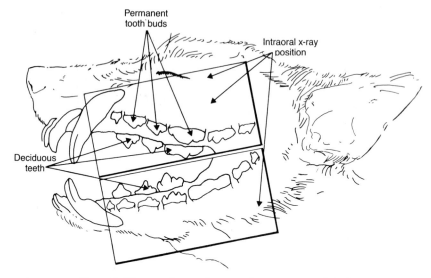

Figure 7. Diagram showing location of permanent tooth buds.

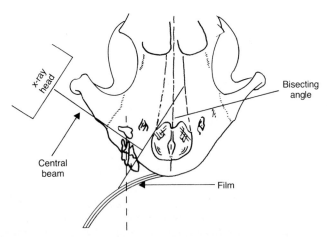

Figure 8. Anterior view of x-ray head position and film placement for lateral radiograph using bisecting angle technique.

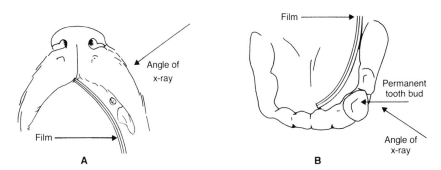

Figure 9. *A*, Maxilla. *B*, Mandible.

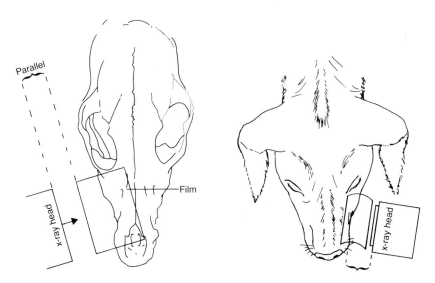

Figure 10. Placement of film and x-ray head to prevent superimposition of structures on lateral views. *A*, Superior position of film and x-ray. *B*, X-ray head parallel to intraoral film.

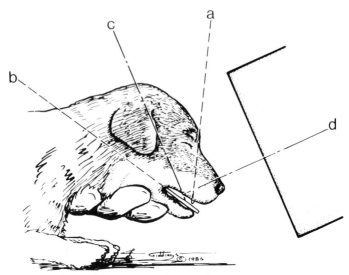

Figure 11. Positioning for anterior maxillary occlusal view in a tranquilized puppy. a = long axis of tooth (canine). b = film plane. c = bisecting angle. d = x-ray beam.

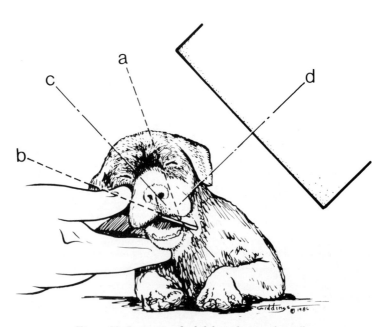

Figure 12. Positioning for left lateral view of maxilla.

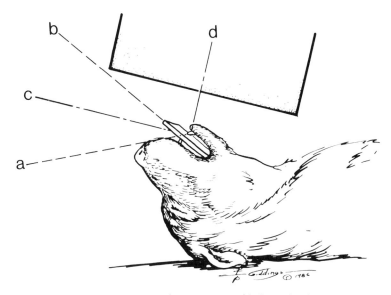

Figure 13. Positioning for anterior mandibular occlusal view.

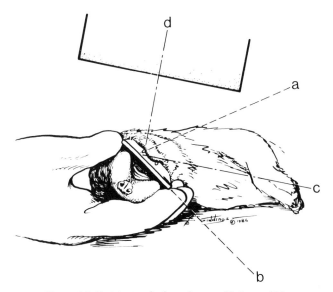

Figure 14. Positioning for lateral view of left mandible.

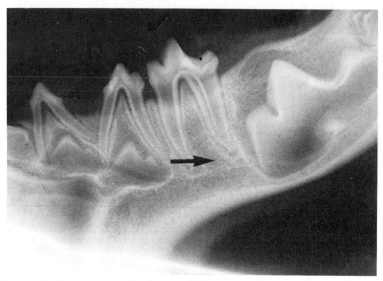

Figure 15. Lateral view of right mandible. Circle shows missing fourth premolar permanent tooth bud.

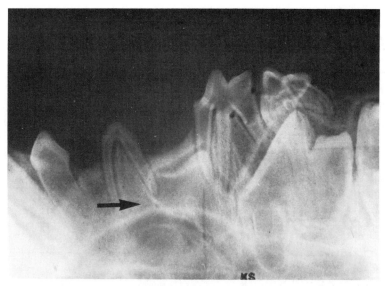

Figure 16. Lateral view of left maxilla. Circle shows missing second premolar permanent tooth bud.

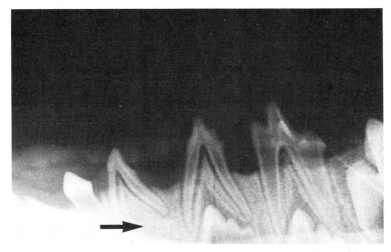

Figure 17. Poor film placement for lateral view, but it still shows absence of permanent tooth bud.

numorphan, subcutaneously, prior to the procedure. A well-tranquilized puppy expedites this procedure. A ventral recumbency is used for the upper arch and a dorsal recumbency is used for the lower arch. The first exposure is an occlusal view of the upper anterior teeth (Figs. 5 and 11) followed by an upper right and left lateral exposure (Figs. 8, 9, and 12). Position the occlusal film as shown in the diagram just caudal to the puppy canine to be sure of radiographing all the permanent tooth buds (Figs. 6 and 7). Radiograph the lower arch in a like manner with the puppy placed in dorsal recumbency. Film is placed in the mouth, and the lower anterior dentition is radiographed as in Figure 13. Film is positioned in the mouth in the right and left mandibular quadrants immediately caudal to the puppy canine, as seen in Figure 14, and radiographed. Follow the same bisecting angle technique and x-ray head position as followed for the maxillary radiography. Note, again, that the technique values are 55 to 65 kVp and 8 to 10 MAS, at 2/5 to 1/2 seconds and a 10-inch focal distance for a dental x-ray and an approximate time for the standard veterinary x-ray is 60 kVp and 100 MAS, at 1/20 second with a 10-inch focal distance. The films are developed in a standard or portable x-ray tank. Multiple dental film clips and a film holder (10 to 14 clips on one holder) will allow for six films, which is the total number needed for one puppy, to be developed at one time in a standard developing tank. A portable developing tank can hold but one x-ray film at a time on a single film clip. The x-ray can be developed in 1 to 1 1/2 minutes with the use of the portable developing tank and a rapid developer and fixer solution. Follow the manufacturer's instructions carefully to obtain the optimum results when using the portable developing tank and rapid developer.

Figures 15 and 16 are examples of good technique. The circle overlay indicates a missing premolar (lower right 4th premolar in Fig. 15, and upper left 2nd premolar in Fig. 16). Figure 17 shows poor film placement and elongation, but it is still readable; again, we wish only to ascertain if tooth buds are present.

REFERENCE

1. O'Brien, R. C.: Dental radiography: An introduction for dental hygienists and assistants. 3:1977.

Animal Dentistry
College of Veterinary Medicine and Biomedical Sciences
Colorado State University
Fort Collins, Colorado 80523

Dentistry   0195–5616/86 $0.00 + .20

Periodontal Disease

Etiology and Pathogenesis

Ben Colmery, III, D.V.M., and Patricia Frost, D.V.M.†*

Periodontal disease is the number-one cause for the early loss of teeth in dogs and cats, as it is in human beings. The great number of toothless Poodles, Yorkshire Terriers, Bichon Frises, Chihuahuas, and so on is due to the effects of periodontal disease. As veterinarians, we are in a position to do something about this situation and improve the oral health of countless dogs and cats. Although many definitions of periodontal disease exist, the most revealing is "gingivitis that has been neglected." It is the effect of long-term gingivitis with its evolution into periodontal disease that concerns the practitioner.

In 1967, Bell studied 600 dogs and found that 75 per cent of the cases had periodontal disease.[1] Hamp et al. in 1984 studied 162 dogs that were anesthetized or euthanatized and found that 83.3 per cent had dental deposits, with 63.6 per cent having periodontitis.[7] When these dogs were grouped by age, periodontitis was found in more than 80 per cent of the animals 6 years of age and older. A 1982 study done by Von Schlup in Bern, Switzerland, found that 57.5 per cent of 200 cats studied had some form of periodontal disease.[15] There are many factors predisposing and contributing to this incidence. The following is a discussion of some of the factors in the adult animal that play a major role in the development of periodontal disease.

OVERCROWDING

In general, this is a much greater problem in small-breed dogs and brachycephalic dogs than in large dogs and mesacephalic or

*Westarbor Animal Hospital, Ann Arbor, Michigan
†Veterinary Dental Service, Roosevelt Roads Naval Station, Ceiba, Puerto Rico

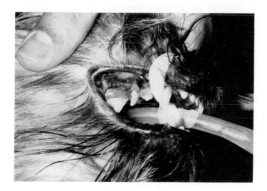

Figure 1. Rotation of maxillary third premolar in a Yorkshire Terrier.

dolicephalic dogs. Usually the smaller dogs tend to have teeth too big for their dental arches, resulting in overlapping of tooth crowns or 90 degree rotation. In brachycephalic skulls, the third, second, and sometimes the first maxillary premolars are rotated (Fig. 1). These deviations from normal predispose the teeth to food entrapment, which then contributes to plaque and calculus formation. In pet dogs with nonmotivated owners, extraction of affected teeth will solve the problem; however, aggressive periodontal therapy and home care will maintain these teeth in those dogs with motivated owners. Breeders of small-breed dogs must be counseled on the problems of tooth size in dental arches and taught what to look for. In general, it is much easier to change skeleton size rather than tooth size. Thus, breeders may have to rethink their long-range breeding goals. Brachycephalic animals will be plagued with tooth rotation and crowding as long as the skull type exists. The preceding information applies to the feline species as well.

MOUTH BREATHING

Brachycephalic dogs are much more likely to have periodontal problems due to mouth breathing than dogs with other skull types. Mouth breathing results from stenotic nares and/or elongated soft palates. Both conditions cause the animal to rely on an open mouth for air exchange, creating gingiva that is continually being dried out. This constant drying acts as a mechanical irritant, creating a gingivitis that predisposes the animal to gingival hypertrophy and periodontitis. Thus, examination of all animals when under general anesthesia should include assessment of the nares and soft palate for possible surgical intervention.

MALOCCLUSIONS

The true occlusal pattern is a scissors bite. The only teeth in the dog designed for occlusal contact are the table surfaces of the mandibular first, second, and third molars and maxillary first and second molars. The rest of the teeth in the mouth should not contact each other. In cases of pathologic malocclusion, teeth striking opposing teeth results in constant trauma. Not only do the crowns wear abnormally, but the periodontal fibers resorb and inflammation ensues. This process usually takes many years, and when the teeth are ultimately lost, severe oral destruction occurs. The best recommendation for the pet owner is to either orthodontically move the teeth when ethically and medically appropriate or surgically extract the teeth. To ignore the malocclusions is not fair to the animal.

DIET

Numerous studies indicate the importance of the type of diet offered the animal and the status of the oral cavity. The best type of food is the dry type, which offers resistance therapy. It maintains periodontal tone, and the abrasiveness of the food scrapes off plaque when chewed dry. This is especially true in the cat. As with all rules, there is always the exception. The authors have examined the oral cavities of racing sled dogs in Fairbanks, Alaska, and found them to be in superior condition despite the fact that these dogs are fed a wet, mush-type diet. The dogs are bred for health, speed, and temperament, rather than beauty. Also, the breeders do not breed immunodeficient animals. The severity of the winters kills the weak, so what is left are structurally healthy animals. Healthy, immunocompetent animals are obviously more apt to tolerate wider ranges of care and their immune systems are better able to cope with all sorts of problems.

BEHAVIOR

Boredom is a significant problem in many animals. Fence, rock, and bone chewing are ways dogs fill empty time, and this destruction compromises the health of their mouths. Fractured teeth with resultant endodontic disease as well as partial tooth avulsions and gingival lacerations are common in their mouths. Substitute objects such as rawhide bones or various synthetic bones are preferable over boulders and knuckle bones. Dogs who are fence chewers will continue to suffer from increased crown wear as long as the behavior

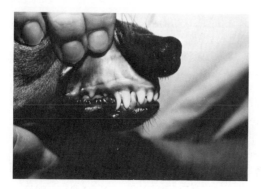

Figure 2. Retained deciduous canine with accumulated plaque and debris between the teeth.

persists. If the owners are unable to find alternative care methods, fence chewers will ultimately break their teeth, necessitating endodontic therapy. Obviously, this is a difficult issue without single solutions.

Equally devastating are electrical burns in cats' mouths from electric cord chewing. Hiding electric cords from curious cats can be a challenge. Chemical burns from household cleaning agents and irritant burns from poisonous houseplants can be a problem if pet owners are unwilling or unable to prevent them.

DEVELOPMENTAL DEFECTS

One of the greatest contributing factors to malocclusions and also periodontal disease is the retention of deciduous teeth (Fig. 2). While common in small breed dogs, it is observed in all species of animals. This problem is easily dealt with by simply extracting the retained tooth. The best time to do the procedure is at the earliest hint of retention. Often, deciduous teeth are extracted prophylactically in breeds with the problem. Besides malocclusions, retained teeth promote food entrapment between the crowns, with resultant periodontitis.

Other developmental defects such as micrognathia, cleft palate, and polydontia are dealt with in an appropriate manner. The goal is to have the correct number of teeth in their correct positions without any interference. Each situation requires a perception of function, with the therapeutic goal to maintain normal function and easy home care.

METABOLIC AND SYSTEMIC DISEASE

Enamel hypoplasia, while considered a developmental defect, is usually the result of any febrile disease of young dogs during the enamel-forming age of their permanent dentition. The result of enamel hypoplasia is exposure of the more porous dentinal layers. The dentin aids in accumulation of plaque and calculus by providing a surface for easy attachment. Therapy involves either aggressive dental prophylaxis and home care or use of the various dental restoratives to create a smoother surface. If ignored, significant periodontitis ultimately results.

Other metabolic and systemic diseases may have oral manifestations. Uremic animals usually have oral ulcerations such as buccal cavity ulcers. This is especially evident in animals with congenital renal hypoplasia. Hypothyroid animals sometimes have concurrent ulcerative stomatitis. Cats positive for feline leukemia virus often have severe periodontal problems, and pemphigus animals usually have refractory periodontal disease.

PATHOPHYSIOLOGY

The preceding are some of the factors that influence whether or not a particular dog is going to develop periodontal disease. By reviewing the etiology and pathogenesis of periodontal disease, we can understand the treatment necessary to prevent and control the disease.

Periodontal disease is defined as the disease and progressive inflammation and destruction of the periodontium. The periodontium consists of those structures surrounding and supporting the tooth: the gingiva, cementum, dentogingival junction, periodontal ligament, and alveolar process. The area in which this disease process occurs is the crevicular groove. Considering the normal anatomy of the tooth and periodontium in the normal dog, the crevicular groove (gingival sulcus) is very shallow, only 1 to 2 mm deep. The free gingival margin has a fine, tapered point that fits closely against the enamel surface. There are no dental deposits on the tooth. There is no gingival swelling or reddening, and the gingival surface is a glistening pink and firm (Fig. 3). Neutrophils pass freely from the gingival tissue through the junctional epithelium into the gingival sulcus, as part of the local defense system. This situation changes as plaque accumulates on the tooth surface. Plaque consists of soft bacterial deposits that adhere to the surface of the tooth, which is covered by a thin, acellular membrane called the pellicle. As these microorganisms from the saliva attach to the pellicle and multiply, they can form a continuous deposit in 2 to 5 days. After 10 days without oral hygiene, the plaque deposit reaches its maximal thickness. After this time, new deposits counterbalance any amounts that are worn off by frictional forces (Fig. 4).

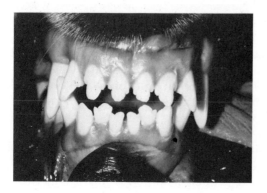

Figure 3. Appearance of normal gingiva and periodontium in a young dog before the accumulation of dental deposits.

Initially, the bacteria found in plaque are streptococci and straight rods. As the development of gingivitis takes place, the flora changes from predominantly nonmotile, gram-positive, aerobic coccoid microbial flora to a more motile, gram-negative rod-shaped anaerobic flora. This change can occur within 2 weeks when plaque is allowed to accumulate. The most common bacteria found in supra- and subgingival plaque are *Bacteroides melaninogenicus* and *Fusobacterium nucleatum*. Supragingival plaque has been described as containing predominantly gram-positive bacteria; subgingival plaque contains predominantly gram-negative bacteria. Spirochetes have also been found by various researchers in plaque deposits. With this accumulation of plaque on the tooth surface and in the gingival sulcus, several processes take place. The gingival sulcus is enlarged, allowing for the accumulaiton of plaque and debris. Numerous interactions between the microbial flora are going on, causing an inflammatory reaction of the surrounding gingival tissues. The release of bacterial endotoxins, enzymes, and antigen-antibody reactions has been proposed to be the initiating factor of this inflammatory process. There is an increase in the numbers of neutrophils moving into the

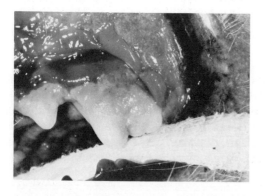

Figure 4. Accumulated plaque and debris on the buccal surface of maxillary premolars.

gingival sulcus and an increase in the morphology and permeability of the vessels in the gingival tissues. The gingival margin becomes reddened and swollen. Gingival fluid is increased, and a cellular infiltrate is formed. This cellular infiltrate in dogs is made up predominantly of plasma cells. As the amount of plaque increases and becomes mineralized to form calculus, which collects more plaque, this inflammatory process increases. The junctional epithelium becomes ulcerated, and the cellular infiltrate adjacent to the pocket epithelium increases. The gingival sulcus becomes deepened as the inflammatory process starts the destruction of the periodontal ligaments, and true periodontal disease is present. As these destructive processes occur and the periodontal pocket deepens, more material is collected as the gingival tissue continues to swell and move away from the tooth surface. Frequently, in dogs there is a greater recession of the gingival tissue without deep pocket formation. As the process advances to the level of the alveolar bone, osteoclastic resorption of bone, cementum, and dentin occurs. When half of the vertical length of the alveolus is lost, the tooth will be lost. After loss of the tooth, which is now acting more like a foreign body, the alveolus can drain and fill in with granulation tissue. This entire process occurs over several years, which is the reason many dogs are not seen for clinical dental problems until they are over 5 years of age; it also accounts for the increased incidence in older dogs. These processes may occur in only a few teeth, in several teeth at a time, or involve only one root of a multiroot tooth. Generally, the premolars are the first teeth to become involved and the first to be lost. Any one dog can have one or more stages of periodontal disease in its mouth.

Clinically, the first signs are an increase in halitosis as the plaque accumulates on the tooth surface. If an explorer is run over the surface of the tooth, plaque can be removed. As the plaque becomes mineralized to form calculus, these deposits are seen supragingivally as a thin build-up of yellow-brown material at the gingival margin (Fig. 5). Subgingival calculus can be seen if the free gingival margin is pushed up; it is usually dark brown with a harder consistency. As the calculus and plaque deposits accumulate and the gingival tissues become more inflamed, a marginal gingivitis is seen. There is reddening and swelling, with a rounding of the free gingival margin and increased bleeding of the gingiva. An inflammatory exudate will be present in the gingival sulcus. As periodontitis is initiated, the gingivitis will be more severe. The surface of the marginal gingiva becomes hyperplastic and cauliflower-like. There is a distinct line of demarcation between the normal tissue and the diseased tissue. The remaining attached gingiva becomes narrower as the hyperplastic tissue enlarges. Pus will be present around the

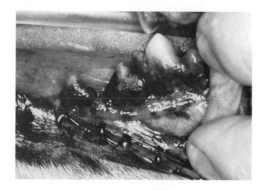

Figure 5. Supragingival calculus accumulation with gingival recession.

exposed tooth root and increased tooth mobility can be seen (Fig. 6). Periodontal pockets, if present, can be diagnosed with a probe. Ulcerations of the buccal mucosa are often seen opposite sites of calculus accumulation. Radiographically, there will be an increased erosion of the alveolar process with a loss of bone height. Areas with the largest accumulation of hyperplastic tissue are correlated with increased pocket depth. As the disease progresses, the animal may show signs of difficulty in eating, anorexia, severe halitosis, pawing at the mouth, or bleeding from the mouth. An animal with a low-grade infection may present with episodes of hepatitis, kidney disease, or gastrointestinal disease from the periodic bacteremia that can occur during eating.

Periodontal disease can present in several forms. It is important to recognize and understand what is happening with each of these forms in order to apply the proper treatment. Periodontal disease may present as gingival recession with exposure of root surface. This recession can be so severe that the teeth will nearly be exfoliated, but there will be no pocket formation. The small periodontal pocket

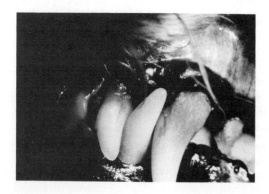

Figure 6. Severe periodontal disease with gingival recession, pyorrhea, and tooth mobility.

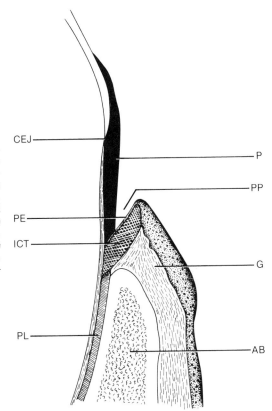

Figure 7. Diagrammatic representation of gingival recession without pocket formation. The gingiva (G) has retracted beyond the cementoenamel junction (CEJ). Plaque (P) covers the crown and exposed root surface and fills the shallow periodontal pocket (PP). Pocket epithelium (PE) covers the infiltrated connective tissue (ICT). AB = alveolar bone. PL = periodontal ligament fibers.

is filled with plaque. The pocket epithelium is ulcerated and covers the infiltrated connective tissue. The gingiva is swollen and reddened, with a distinct line of demarcation between normal and diseased tissue (Fig. 7).

Periodontal disease may also present as the type of pocket formation seen more commonly in humans. The gingiva is swollen and reddened, but the free gingival margin remains at the cementoenamel junction. A deep periodontal pocket is formed with loss of alveolar bone. This pocket is filled with microbial plaque to the depth of the pocket. The alveolar bone loss can either be horizontal or vertical. With horizontal bone loss, the depth of the pocket stays above the level of the alveolar bone; this is called a suprabony pocket (Fig. 8). If the pocket depth goes below the level of the alveolar bone, this is termed an intrabony pocket (Fig. 9). The demarcation between normal and diseased tissues may be more obscure, and there is a broad zone of infiltrated connective tissue.

A third presentation of the disease is often seen in dogs with advanced periodontitis. The lesion will be fiery red with cauliflower-

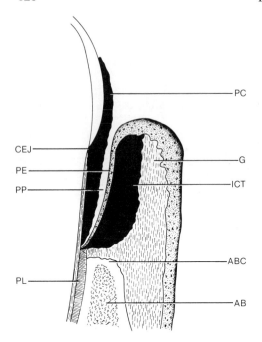

Figure 8. Diagrammatic representation of a suprabony periodontal pocket. There is a deep periodontal pocket (*PP*) filled with plaque and calculus (*PC*) that has destroyed the periodontal ligament fibers (*PL*) and alveolar bone (*AB*). The alveolar bone crest (*ABC*) remains apical to the depth of the pocket. There is a broad zone of infiltrated connective tissue (*ICT*) covered by ulcerated pocket epithelium (*PE*). *CEJ* = cementoenamel junction. *G* = gingiva.

Figure 9. Intrabony pocket formation. In this situation, the destruction of the periodontal ligament fibers (*PL*) has advanced ahead of the alveolar bone crest (*ABC*). The periodontal pocket (*PP*) is filled with plaque (*P*). *ICT* = infiltrated connective tissue. *PE* = pocket epithelium. *G* = gingiva. *CEJ* = cementoenamel junction.

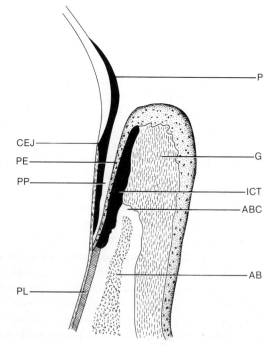

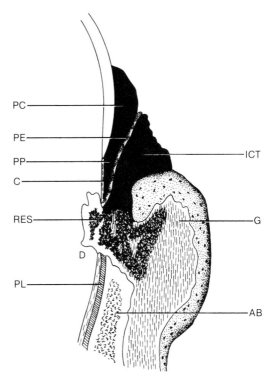

Figure 10. Diagrammatic representation of advanced periodontitis in a dog. There is hyperplastic gingiva (G) covering areas of resorption (RES) of the cementum (C) and dentin (D). There is a large amount of infiltrated connective tissue (ICT) that may protrude out of the shallow periodontal pocket (PP). The pocket is filled with plaque and calculus (PC). CEJ = cementoenamel junction. AB = alveolar bone. PL = periodontal ligament. PE = pocket epithelium.

like hyperplastic gingiva. This is an active and destructive situation, with accumulation of pus, calculus, and debris in the periodontal pocket. The infiltrated connective tissue is large and may extend beyond the level of normal gingiva. There is extensive loss of alveolar bone, and resorption of the cementum and dentin can occur (Fig. 10).

Periodontal disease in cats has not been studied extensively, but it seems that the disease process is fairly similar to that in dogs. In the studies that have been done, the premolars and molars are the most commonly affected, although the incisors are most frequently lost early. The hyperplastic presentation of periodontitis is not seen that frequently. The cat does have an interesting presentation of periodontal disease, however—that of the subgingival resorptive lesion (neck lesions) seen at or below the cementoenamel junction (Fig. 11). These lesions are found in 20 to 30 per cent of the cats studied and occur mainly in the premolars and molars on the buccal surface. They have been found on the lingual surfaces and in the canine teeth. The exact mechanism of these resorptive lesions has not been determined, but they are not carious lesions, as was first thought. There is an osteoclastic resorptive process with

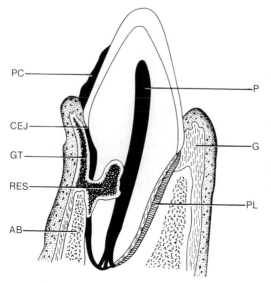

PC

CEJ

GT

RES

AB

P

G

PL

Figure 11. Diagrammatic representation of an advanced subgingival resorptive lesion in a cat. Area of resorption (*RES*) may extend to the pulp (*P*). The defect may be covered by granulation tissue (*GT*), plaque, and calculus (*PC*). *CEJ* = cementoenamel junction. *G* = gingiva. *AB* = alveolar bone. *PL* = periodontal ligament.

some evidence of repair with secondary dentin. These lesions occur at the cementoenamel junction and are often covered with calculus or the gingival margin and will not be seen until the subgingival area is probed with an explorer. In many cases, the root resorption can be quite extensive, leading to fracture of the tooth with retention of the remaining root. Whether or not these lesions are a result of the periodontal disease process in cats has yet to be determined. They have been found in younger cats without obvious signs of periodontitis. An increase in these lesions has been associated with cats that are on an exclusive liver diet. The lesions may or may not be painful to the animal, probably depending upon the severity of resorption close to the pulp tissue. One or more teeth in any one cat may be affected. When these lesions are extensive, it makes for difficult extraction, because the weakened root fractures so easily

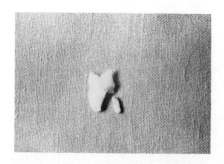

Figure 12. Extracted mandibular molar from a cat with a subgingival resorptive lesion leading to a fracture of the caudal root. Remaining root tip must also be removed.

(Fig. 12). If these resorptive lesions are found early, the tooth can be preserved by doing a restorative procedure to fill the defect.

TREATMENT PLANNING

In order to plan treatment and advise the client as to cost and prognosis, it is often helpful to categorize the animals into Group I (mild), Group II (moderate), or Group III (severe). With periodontal disease, prevention is the best medicine. Routine dental prophylaxis consisting of scaling, subgingival curettage, root planing, if necessary, and polishing, with instructions on home care, can preserve the oral health of the animal. The frequency of these treatments will depend on the individual animal, the ability of the owner to apply home-care treatment, and the motivation of the owner. Usually every 6 to 12 months will be optimum to maintain healthy teeth and interrupt the periodontal disease process. With dogs and cats that are on a regular dental prophylaxis program, there will be minimal calculus build-up and the treatment usually only takes 20 to 30 minutes. These animals would be Group I cases. The time spent to treat these animals will be short; they usually won't need any further treatment, until the next visit, unless there are other dental abnormalities found on inspection. The cost to the owner will be less, and the prognosis is good.

Group II dogs have more extensive involvement with increased amounts of calculus and mild to moderate periodontitis in one or more teeth. Usually the teeth are still solidly attached and either have gingival recession or mild pocket formation (4 to 6 mm). Besides scaling and polishing, subgingival curettage and root planing are required in these cases to remove all the subgingival calculus and plaque and remove the ulcerated pocket epithelium and granulation tissue to allow the gingival tissues to return to normal. Inadequate removal of subgingival plaque leaves the inflammatory nidus present, and although the teeth look cleaner, the disease process will continue to deepen the pockets. After treatment of these cases, there is a reduction in the amount of swelling and reddness of the gum tissue, with subsequent elimination of mild pockets. The prognosis for these teeth is good, particularly if the gingival tissues respond well to the initial therapy. Follow-up home care and more frequent dental prophylaxis visits may be necessary to retain the improved status. If the disease process has gone on for some time, there may be some residual fibrosis of the gingiva that will not change and may require gingival surgery.

Group III animals have moderate to severe periodontitis. They will present with hyperplastic gingiva, deep pockets (6 to 9 mm), severe gingival recession with tooth mobility, pyorrhea, and excessive dental deposits. Group III animals are often older, and a thorough work-up before dental procedures are started should be done to evalute function of the heart, liver, and kidneys. These cases will require more than one visit if severely affected teeth are to be preserved. The time required to complete the treatment will be greater, as will the cost to the client. Tooth mobility should be evaluated first. Any teeth that are readily moved should be noted and extracted. The remaining teeth should be treated as in Group II cases. The teeth should again be checked for mobility, and any questionable teeth removed if the owner is not willing to have further periodontal surgical procedures done. Extraction of mobile or hopelessly involved teeth is necessary because these teeth will act as foreign bodies, and removal allows the remaining dentition to respond better to periodontal treatment. Tooth mobility should be checked in all patients with clinical signs of periodontitis. A tooth in which less than one third of the root structure is surrounded by healthy alveolar bone is hopeless and should be extracted. Teeth that are critical to the dog's function that have deep pockets, root exposure, or bony defects can be preserved with additional periodontal surgical techniques, adequate home care, and frequent follow-up visits. Two to three weeks should be given before re-evaluation for periodontal surgery to allow the gingival tissues to respond to the initial treatment.

Scaling, polishing, root planing, and subgingival curettage are all necessary steps in the treatment of more severe cases of periodontal disease to remove the local initiating factors of the inflammatory process. When the gingival tissues have returned to a more healthy state, the success of periodontal surgery will be greater.

When cases are presented with more severe periodontal disease and the client wishes to do what is necessary to preserve the teeth, several other procedures may be necessary to remove deep pockets and slow down the disease process. These procedures are gingivectomy, gingivoplasty, and gingival flaps. The prognosis for these teeth is guarded, but with these additional surgical procedures, conscientious home care, and more frequent visits for dental proplylaxis, the teeth can function for some time.

TREATMENT PROCEDURES

Treatment procedures and home care are described in the following article ("Periodontal Disease: Therapy and Prevention").

MEDICAL THERAPY

Topical cleaning agents such as Gingival are excellent plaque controllers. Obviously, to be effective they have to be applied to the

Table 1. *Aerobic Culture and Sensitivity Tests from 97 Canine Oral Cavities*

ORGANISM	NO. CULTURES PRESENT	% TOTAL CULTURES*	Drug	No. Times Tested	% Effect
Pasteurella multocida	41	42	Cephalothin	9	100
			Chloramphenicol	35	100
			Tetracycline	19	100
			Erythromycin	17	100
			Ampicillin	19	84
Staphylococcus aureus	33	34	Gentamicin	15	100
			Kanamycin	9	100
			Methicillin	3	100
			Cephalothin	6	100
			Nitrofurantoin	5	100
			Chloramphenicol	29	93
			Erythromycin	24	92
Moroxella sp.	21	22	Chloramphenicol	13	100
			Gentamicin	11	100
			Nitroflurantoin	7	100
			Tetracycline	7	100
			Ampicillin	11	91
Beta-hemolytic streptococcus	19	20	Chloramphenicol	16	100
			Erythromycin	13	100
			Penicillin	16	100
			Lincomycin	16	87
			Ampicillin	8	87

The ANTIBIOTIC SENSITIVITY heading spans the Drug, No. Times Tested, and % Effect columns.

*Most cultures had more than one organism present.

teeth. The owners must understand that the animal is dependent upon the owner to continue using these products.

Antibiotics are used short-term during acute gingival flare-ups and presurgically to minimize iatrogenic septicemias caused by dental manipulations. Table 1 shows the results of a study at Michigan State University where bacterial populations and their antibiotic sensitivities were studied from the oral cavities of dogs with gingivitis.

In animals with severe immune-mediated stomatitis and gingivitis, plaque control is an absolute necessity. These animals are usually borderline hypothyroid and clinically feel better with thyroid replacement therapy. Immunomodulation with products like Staph Lysate helps as adjunct therapy in animals with profound staphylococcal involvement. Other drugs that are found to be helpful are listed in Table 2.

SUMMARY

In conclusion, the oral cavity represents a complex dynamic state of evolving physiology from health into disease. Although this

Table 2

COMPOUND	INDICATIONS	DOSAGE	ROUTE
Metronidazole	Ulcerative stomatitis, gingivitis, periodontitis	50 mg /kg once a day	Oral
Ketoconazole	Oral candidiasis, systemic fungal infections	10 mg/kg as single or divided dose	Oral
Chlorhexidine	Periodontal disease, oral cleansing	0.2% solution	As oral rinse or toothbrush solution
Carbamide peroxide	Plaque control	Q.S.	Topical
Benzathine penicillin/procaine penicillin	Gingivitis, periodontitis	30,000 units/lb	Intramuscular
Staphage lysate	Immune-mediated stomatitis	Weekly intervals .1 cc ID, then add .1 cc weekly to .5 cc, then increase weekly intervals to bimonthly to monthly	First dose ID, then all others subcutaneously

process is slow, it is usually inevitable. Fortunately, the majority of animals respond to veterinary intervention and owner motivation. There are a few animals, however, whose periodontal problems are refractory to treatment, and wholesale tooth extraction is the only viable option.

REFERENCES

1. Bell, A. F.: Dental disease in the dog. J. Small Anim. Pract., 6:421–428, 1967.
2. Colmery, B.: Dentistry. In Bojrab, J. M. (ed.): Pathophysiology in Small Animal Surgery. Philadelphia, Lea & Febiger, 1981.
3. Eisenmenger, E., and Zetner, K.: Veterinary Dentistry. Edition 1. Philadelphia, Lea & Febiger, 1985.
4. Gad, T.: Periodontal disease in dogs. 1. Clinical investigations. J. Periodont. Res., 3(4):268, 1968.
5. Grant, D., Stern, J., and Everett, F.: Orban's Periodontics. Edition 4. St. Louis, Missouri, C. V. Mosby Co., 1972.
6. Hamp. S. E., and Lindberg, R.: Histopathology of spontaneous periodontitis in dogs. J. Periodont. Res., 12(1):46, 1977.
7. Hamp, S. E., Olsson, K., Farso-Madsen, K., et al.: A microscopic and radiologic investigation of dental diseases of the dog. Vet. Radiol., 25:86–92, 1984.
8. Harvey, C. E.: Veterinary Dentistry. 1. Philadelphia, W. B. Saunders Co., 1985.
9. Hull, P. S., Soames, J. V., and Davies, R. M.: Periodontal disease in a Beagle dog colony. J. Comp. Pathol., 84(2):143, 1974.
10. Lindhe, J., Hamp. S. E., and Loe, H.: Plaque-induced periodontal disease in Beagle

    dogs. A 4-year clinical, roentgenographic and histometrical study. J. Periodont. Res.,
    10(5):243, 1975.
11. Page, R. C., and Schroeder, H. E.: Periodontitis in Man and Other Animals: A
    Comparative Review. New York, S. Karger, 1982.
12. Page, R. C., and Schroeder, H. E.: Spontaneous chronic periodontitis in adult dogs: A
    clinical and histopathological survey. J. Periodontol., *52*(2):60, 1981.
13. Reichart, P. A., et al.: Periodontal disease in the domestic cat: A histologic study. J.
    Periodont. Res., *19*:67–75, 1984.
14. Ross, D. L.: Veterinary dentistry. *In* Ettinger, S. J. (ed.): Textbook of Veterinary Internal
    Mecicine. Volume 1. Philadelphia, W. B. Saunders Co., 1975.
15. Von Schlup, D.: Epidemiologische und morphologische Untersuchungen am Katzen-
    gebiB I. Mitteilung: Epidemiologische Untersuchungen. Kleinterpraxis, *27*:87–94,
    1982.
16. Von Schlup, D., Stich, H.: Epidemiologische und morphologische Untersuchungen am
    KatzengebiB II. Mitteilung: Morphologische Untersuchungen der "neck lesions."
    Kleinterpraxis, *27*:179–188, 1982.
17. Schneck, G. W., and Osborn, J. W.: Neck lesions in the teeth of cats. Vet. Rec.,
    99(6):100. 7, 1976.
18. Shafer, W., Hine, M., and Levy, B.: Textbook of Oral Pathology. Edition 3. Philadelphia,
    W. B. Saunders Co., 1974.
19. Sorensen, W. P., and Ramfjord, S. P.: Periodontal disease in the Beagle dog: A cross
    sectional clinical study. J. Periodont. Res., *15*(4):380, 1980.
20. Studer, E., and Stapley, R. B.: The role of dry foods in maintaining healthy teeth and
    gums in the cat. Vet. Med. Small Anim. Clin., 1124–1126, 1973.

Westarbor Animal Hospital
6011 Jackson Road
Ann Arbor, Michigan 48103

0195–5616/86 $0.00 + .20

Periodontal Disease

Therapy and Prevention

*B. Jean Hawkins, M.S., D.V.M.**

Tholen, in his text, *Concepts of Veterinary Dentistry*, states, "Periodontal disease is present . . . in approximately 85 per cent of all small animals . . . more than six years old."[15] The procedures for diagnosing and treating periodontal disease are very simple but specific. Basic instrumentation is well within the range, economically, of every practitioner, providing an area of easily expanded services.

Periodontal disease is often an incidental finding during the physical examination and may not be considered clinically important until the disease has led to extreme tooth mobility or tooth loss. Periodontal disease of this degree is generally found in older pets, leading to the erroneous conclusion that is it a geriatric condition. Grove, however, found that gingivitis (reversible change) develops at 1 to 2 years of age and periodontitis (irreversible change) appears at 4 to 6 years of age in the Beagle.[4]

To prevent the development of irreversible changes in the periodontium, *preventive* dental care must be started in the very young pet. This will consist of client education in home-care techniques and the benefits of regular veterinary dental prophylaxis for the pet.

THE DENTAL PROPHYLAXIS

The dental prophylaxis is generally not performed as an emergency procedure. A proper physical examination coupled with clinical evaluation of the patient should be conducted and evaluated prior

*Orchard Animal Clinic, Boise, Idaho

to anesthesia.[15] Many times, borderline changes will occur in serum chemistries, indicating the onset of a disease process. Also, some systemic diseases such as chronic nephritis, hyperparathyroidism, diabetes mellitus, and immune-mediated disorders may influence the severity of periodontal disease.[15] The patient should be assessed, existing conditions treated, and the dental prophylaxis scheduled when the patient improves or stabilizes, often in only 2 to 3 weeks.

THE DENTAL RECORD

A dental chart should be kept in the patient's record. Prior to any dental procedure, basic information such as bite; degree of periodontal disease present; missing, fractured, discolored, maligned, supernumerary, worn, or retained deciduous teeth; and abnormalities of soft tissue should be recorded.

THE BASIC HAND INSTRUMENT

Hand instruments have three distinct sections: the handle, the shank, and the working end. The handle may be pencil thin but is more comfortable to grip if slightly enlarged. The shank is either straight or angled one or more times to accommodate working in various mouth areas. The working end denotes the function of the instrument. In a well-designed instrument, the working end is nearly in a straight line with the handle. The instrument may be single-ended (SE) or double-ended (DE). The working ends may be mirror images or complementary in use.

A modified pen grasp is the most effective method for holding a hand instrument. The thumb and forefinger are placed at the junction of the handle and shank. The pad of the index finger rests at the junction of the shank and working end. The ring finger is placed firmly on the closest surface to the tooth being scaled to serve as a fulcrum. To develop the skill necessary to control the instrument tip, a small circle is drawn and the ring finger positioned in the center. A pencil is grasped with the modified pen grasp and the tip moved to inscribe an arc. The objective is to control the instrument tip so that it adapts to the tooth surface, which increases scaling efficiency and decreases iatrogenic gingival trauma.[11]

EXPLORER AND PROBE

The gingivae may exhibit relatively few signs of subgingival calculus; however, accumulations of subgingival calculus within the

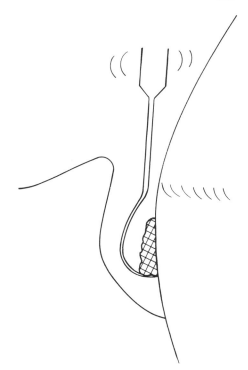

Figure 1. Detecting subgingival calculus.

gingival sulcus can easily be located by using a dental explorer.[11] The thin tip of this instrument, when inserted into the gingival sulcus, allows the operator to tactically sense the presence of irregularities of the cemental surface of the tooth root (Fig. 1). Early detection and removal of subgingival calculus is essential in the prevention and control of periodontal disease. The delicate explorer tip is also used to assess tooth mobility. (The periodontal ligaments provide each tooth with slight normal mobility and shock-absorbing capacity.) Teeth that are noticeably more mobile than adjacent teeth should be evaluated for destructive processes that may necessitate surgery or extraction. Lower incisors may be somewhat mobile, however, because they occasionally share alveoli (the operator should also remain aware of calcium-depleting conditions).

The explorer also provides the operator with a method of evaluating the smoothness of the root surface after periodontal therapy. Undetected or removed subgingival calculus continues to irritate subgingival tissues, and the progess of periodontal disease continues unchecked.

As periodontal disease progresses, changes occur in the gingival sulcus depth.[5] The periodontal probe is used to measure this depth.

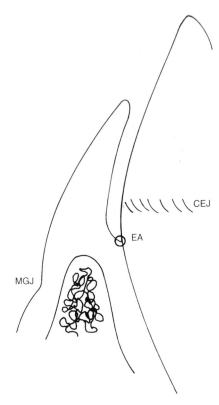

Figure 2. Gingival pocket. *MGJ* = mucogingival junction. *EA* = epithelial attachment. *CEJ* = cementoenamel junction.

The working end of the probe is thin, straight, and calibrated in millimeters (10 to 12 mm total). The probe should be held parallel to the long axis of the tooth and inserted gently into the sulcus until soft-tissue resistance is felt. The normal depth of the gingival sulcus, which encircles each tooth, is 1 to 3 mm. The probe should be gently moved circumferentially within the sulcus to eliminate overlooking pockets.[13] If the probe depth is greater than 3 mm, a gingival or periodontal pocket is usually present. To differentiate between the two, the cementoenamel junction is located with the explorer tip. A gingival pocket (reversible) will have the major portion of tissue coronal to the cementoenamel junction (Fig. 2), whereas the periodontal pocket (irreversible) depth will be primarily apical to the cementoenamel junction (Fig. 3). This determination is important in treating the pocket.

SUPRAGINGIVAL SCALING

Removal of calculus above the gingival margin can be accomplished with hand instruments alone or in combination with me-

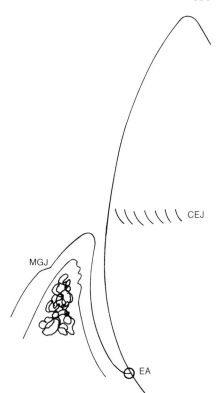

Figure 3. Periodontal pocket.

chanical scalers. An excellent hand scaler for supragingival scaling is a double-ended Jacquette 2Y/3Y. This curved sickle scaler is triangular in cross section and has a modified shank, two cutting edges, and a sharp tip. The curvature provides adequate contact around most curved tooth surfaces, and the sharp tip allows the operator to scale between incisors and crowded teeth.

The most efficient working angle for a scaling hand instrument is between 45 degrees and 90 degrees to the tooth surface.[11] The blade is positioned proximal to the supragingival calculus, the instrument gripped securely with the modified pen grasp, and the ring finger serves as a fulcrum. The blade engages the calculus, and the hand and wrist move together in a pull stroke (pull strokes direct fractured calculus *away* from the gingival sulcus) to fracture the calculus from the tooth surface. One or two strokes with a sharp, properly positioned hand scaler is usually sufficient for gross calculus removal. Lighter pull strokes are used to remove small amounts of calculus from the tooth surface.

SUBGINGIVAL SCALING

Subgingival scaling is the removal of subgingival calculus, usually blackish brown in color, from the root surface. The hand instrument of choice is the double-ended McCall's Curette 13/14. This curette is a semicircle in cross section and has a rounded toe. The curette is held with the modified pen grasp. The cutting edge is angled between 45 degrees and 90 degrees to the tooth surface. A pull, horizontal, or oblique stroke is used for subgingival scaling.[11]

ROOT PLANING AND SUBGINGIVAL CURETTAGE

When subgingival scaling is complete, the soft cemental surface of the tooth root should be smoothed. The curette is employed once again. Twenty to thirty overlapping strokes may be needed to produce a smooth, glassy root surface that is free of irregularities.[11] The explorer should be used to evaluate the surface.

The curette blade is angled against the tissue surface of the gingival sulcus, and digital counterpressure is applied to the gingiva. The curette is pulled firmly against the tissue to remove as much debris and chronically inflamed tissue as possible.

ULTRASONIC SCALING

Ultrasonic scaling is widely used in veterinary dentistry. Ultrasonic scalers can be very effective in removing supragingival and subgingival calculus. Certain principles should be observed during use, however. First, use of ultrasonic scalers creates an accumulation of aerosol and water during use. The patient should be intubated with a cuffed endotracheal tube regardless of the type of anesthesia used.[7] The operator and anyone within 18 inches of the tip should wear a mask. The patient should be positioned with the head tilted down and preferably over a grid to permit proper drainage of fluids and debris. A piece of stockinette pulled over the patient's head will keep the ears out of the working field.

Second, proper adjustment of the ultrasound scaler is necessary for best results. The proper water flow and frequency should be adjusted prior to beginning the scaling procedure. The frequency is reduced to zero and the water flow adjusted so that one to two drops per second fall from the tip. The frequency is gradually increased until all water drops are aerosolized. To check for adequate tuning, a finger is placed lightly against the *side* of the tip for 15 seconds. If no heat is detected, the tuning is correct.

Third, proper use of the instrument is important to prevent iatrogenic trauma to the teeth and gingiva. The ultrasonic tip is moved *lightly* back and forth across the tooth, keeping the tip parallel to the gingival margin. A tooth should not be scaled for more than 15 seconds consecutively.

Special tips have been designed for subgingival scaling. Ultrasonic subgingival calculus removal compares favorably with hand scaling; neither is 100 per cent effective, however. Tactile sensitivity is lost with the ultrasonic scaler, and danger of thermal damage to the tooth and gingivae is present.

ROTARY SCALING

An alternative to ultrasonic scalers is a six-sided bur (Roto-sonic scalers or Roto-Pro) attached to a high-speed dental handpiece. These noncutting burs move vertically and produce vibrations of 20,000 cycles per second.

The rotary burs can be used supragingivally or subgingivally depending on the shape and are effective in root planing 3 to 4 mm deep pockets. They exert a polishing effect on the cleaned surface. Rotary scalers should be used for a short time (15 seconds) with a light, horizontal movement across the tooth surface and a water flow adequate to prevent thermal damage to the tooth.[16]

AIR-TURBINE SCALING

Air-turbine scalers have the advantage of achieving ultrasonic speeds without heat build-up and can be used without a water supply. They may provide a useful alternative scaling technique when portability is desirable, although an air compressor is needed.[15]

DISCLOSING SOLUTION

A disclosing solution should be applied to the teeth to detect any remaining plaque and calculus.

POLISHING

After scaling is complete, the enamel surface still is quite irregular. Polishing cleans the enamel and reduces the surface area to which plaque and calculus can reattach. Also, a smooth surface promotes easier removal of plaque during home-care procedures.

Proper polishing requires the use of a power source, polishing cups, and a flour or very fine grade of polishing compound.[1]

842   B. Jean Hawkins

Flour grade pumice is the least expensive polishing compound. It is mixed with water to form a thin paste. Prepared prophy pastes such as zirconium silicate or silicone dioxide are available in various flavors and may also contain fluoride. To prevent contamination of prepared pastes, a small amount should be removed from the container for use during polishing. Polishing is done with a firm pressure for a short time (15 seconds maximum per tooth). All tooth surfaces are polished.

IRRIGATION

Once the removal of supragingival and subgingival calculus is complete, the gingival sulcus must be flushed to remove any traces of dislodged debris that could serve as a nidus for the reintroduction of infection.

A 30-cc to 60-cc syringe filled with a lavaging solution and fitted with a blunt-tipped 20-gauge needle is satisfactory. Dilute povidone-iodine, 0.2 per cent chlorhexadine, or physiologic sterile saline are adequate for flushing. The use of a water-pressure device is not recommended for irrigation because of the possibility of seeding bacteria into the tissues secondary to the water force.

FLUORIDE TREATMENT

A recent addition to the basic dental prophylaxis is the fluoride treatment. Fluoride serves two purposes: it strengthens the enamel and helps desensitize teeth. After the gingival sulcus is irrigated, the teeth must be dried (a blow-dryer for hair works well). Fluoride gel is applied directly to the teeth, allowed to set undisturbed for 4 minutes, and then rinsed. Calculus dries white on the tooth surface and is occasionally seen. It should be removed.

INSTRUMENT CARE

The ease and efficiency with which a basic dental prophylaxis can be performed depends on good technique and equipment that functions properly.

Hand instruments must be sharpened frequently to maintain the original shape and keep the blade sharp. Not only do dull instruments slow the prophylaxis procedure, they are also inefficient at completely removing calculus. Calculus may actually be burnished to the tooth surface by scaling with dull instruments.

An Arkansas sharpening stone and oil stone oil are needed for sharpening hand instruments.

The instruments must be clean before beginning. A good light source and work bench are helpful when sharpening.

Hand instruments such as the curved sickle scaler and curette can be sharpened using a flat or conical stone. Facial sharpening with the conical stone alone is adequate to maintain a sharp cutting edge *if* the instrument is sharpened frequently. For facial sharpening, the conical stone is held in the working hand and the instrument is positioned, flat surface up, firmly in the other hand. The stone is rotated against the flat surface, moving it with the curve of the instrument to prevent excess pressure and wear against the instrument tip. This is repeated three or four times, and the instrument is checked for sharpness by "scaling" a plastic stick or a fingernail. A sharp cutting edge will "bite" into the surface being scaled with a minimum effort. Sharpening scalers and curettes by other methods may be desirable. These techniques can be found in texts for dental hygienists. Instruments should be stored in an instrument tray to preserve the cutting edges.

Parkes and Kolstad[10] found that the cutting edges of stainless steel periodontal instruments were not dulled by 10 saturated steam sterilization cycles at 250 degrees F.

Ultrasonic and other mechanical instruments will periodically require replacement of the instrument tip. The handpieces should be carefully wiped with a cold sterilizing solution. Manufacturer's suggestions on maintenance should be followed.

PERIODONTAL SURGERY

Periodontal surgery may be necessary in order to properly treat periodontal disease. Surgery is indicated when gingival (reversible, or supra-alveolar) pockets or periodontal (irreversible, or bony involvement) pockets cannot be adequately scaled and root planed (4 to 5 mm deep), when the gingival tissue interferes with home care of the affected tooth or teeth (gingival hyperplasia), or when there is furcation involvement (between tooth roots).[2]

Gingivectomy is the removal of excessive gingival tissue coronal to the cementoenamel junction. This procedure is the method of choice in eliminating hypertrophied or edematous gingivae when there has been no significant apical migration of the epithelial attachment. Before performing a gingivectomy, the surgeon must confirm that 2 mm of attached gingiva will remain postoperatively. Otherwise, another method of treatment should be selected.

The depth of the gingival pocket is measured with the peri-

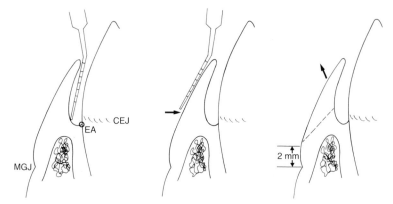

Figure 4. Gingivectomy. *MGJ* = mucogingival junction. *CEJ* = cementoenamel junction. *EA* = epithelial attachment.

odontal probe and is marked on the gingival surface. The tissue is incised so that a smoothly contoured edge and a sulcus depth of no more than 3 mm results. A scalpel or electrosurgical unit is satisfactory (Fig. 4). Bleeding is usually controlled by pressure, although commercial preparations are available.

SIMPLE APICALLY REPOSITIONED FLAP

Flap surgery involves the movement of gingival tissue to allow access to root and osseous structures. It is the method of choice when there is minimal attached gingivae (less than 2 mm) over a pocket area, when there is furcation involvement, or when root resection is deemed necessary.

A simple apically repositioned flap may be adequate for initial flap surgery (Fig. 5). The gingiva is incised 2 to 3 mm lateral to each side of the pocket. The incision may need to be extended into the alveolar mucosa to allow optimum access to the affected area. The tissue is elevated with a very small periosteal elevator and reflected. The root is scaled and root-planed to remove any subgingival calculus. The angular osseous defects that may be in the margin of the alveolar bone are curetted, ronguered, filed, or removed with a dental bur cooled with physiologic sterile saline so that the bony pocket is eliminated. If there is a furcation involvement, more careful bone removal is required and the prognosis is less favorable because of the difficulty in home care. A flap may need to be elevated on the palatal and buccal surfaces for complete access. When debridement is complete, the flap is repositioned. The leading edge of the

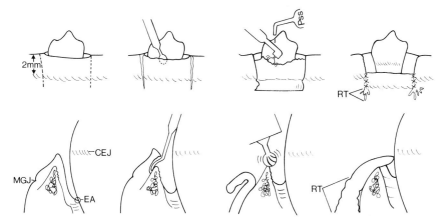

Figure 5. Simple apically repositioned flap. Note the relationship of the mucogingival junction on the flap to that on either side. *MGJ* = mucogingival junction. *CEJ* = cemento-enamel junction. *EA* = epithelial attachment. *RT* = redundant tissue.

flap is positioned to cover the alveolar bone margin. The most apical limit for placement of the leading edge of the flap is the mucogingival junction on either side of the surgical area. There will be slight redundant tissue at the proximal suture line. It will resolve itself.

The flap incisions are closed with simple interrupted 4-0 sutures. Nonabsorbable suture material is less irritating than absorbable material, which sometimes must be removed also. The tissue is held with firm finger pressure for 3 minutes to reduce the space between the flap and alveolar bone. Ideally, a periodontal dressing is applied over the flap to protect the wound, help maintain the flap position, and aid in patient comfort. Practically, the mouth should be flushed with a warm solution of 0.2 per cent chlorhexadine, dilute povidone-iodine, or a salt water solution (if not a cardiac patient) for 5 to 10 days. Good home care is paramount to the success of periodontal surgery.

REVERSE BEVEL FLAP SURGERY

Reverse bevel flap surgery is well described.[3, 5, 8, 15] It requires more surgical technique than a simple apically repositioned flap. The initial horizontal incision removes the gingival margin and, therefore, some of the chronically inflamed lining of the gingival sulcus. This incision is beveled toward the tooth surface, so there will not be an exposed, raw gingival surface upon completion.

The procedure is then the same as the simple apically reposi-tioned flap until closure. To close, the flap is placed in normal

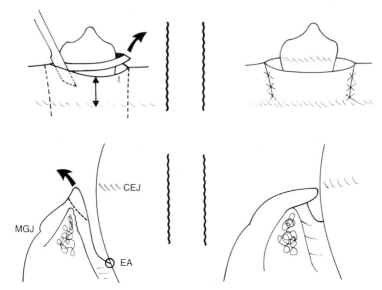

Figure 6. Reverse bevel flap. Note the relationship of the mucogingival junction. Intermediate steps are identical to simple apically repositioned flap. *MGJ* = mucogingival junction. *EA* = epithelial attachment. *CEJ* = cementoenamel junction.

anatomic position and sutured (Fig. 6). Aftercare is the same as for the simple apically repositioned flap.

Many other flap procedures are described.[3, 5, 8, 15] There are applications in veterinary dentistry for most of them at one time or another. However, the majority of cases will no doubt resolve satisfactorily using one of the previously mentioned methods.

Antibiotic therapy should be strongly considered before and for 5 days after the treatment of periodontal pockets.

The periodontal patient should be re-evaluated in 1 to 3 months. Further surgery or extraction of the involved tooth may need to be performed to restore dental health.

HOME CARE

Home care is the most important aspect of veterinary dentistry. The daily removal of plaque minimizes the destructive effects it has on the periodontium and is the prime factor in preventing and controlling periodontal disease.[8]

Client compliance is obviously essential in veterinary dental home care. Thorough client education as to the cause (chronic plaque accumulation on the teeth) and prevention (daily plaque removal and professional dental prophylaxis and periodontal therapy) of periodontal disease are necessary. *Prevention* of permanent damage should be stressed to those clients with young animals (less than 4 years of age), and a regular dental prophylaxis should be scheduled prior to the onset of irreversible changes in the periodontium. The *benefits* of healthy teeth and gingivae such as fresh breath (no "fish breath" odor or halitosis), prevention or elimination of chronic low-grade infections that are inapparent and may cause endocarditis or nephritis, and no tooth loss secondary to periodontal disease[12] should be brought to the client's attention.

Plaque and calculus accumulations are heaviest near salivary gland duct openings—that is, the lingual surface of the lower cheek teeth and buccal surface of upper cheek teeth. The tongue helps keep lingual tooth surfaces somewhat clean. The most critical area for brushing of the pet's teeth, therefore, is the buccal surface of the upper cheek teeth, where the parotid and zygomatic gland duct openings are located (upper P4 and M2, respectively). The pet should be assessed for problems such as existing gingivitis, periodontitis (especially when deep pockets are present), and overcrowded or malaligned teeth. These areas should receive special attention during brushing.

The mechanical effect of toothbrushing is the significant factor in plaque removal. Special instruction should be given to the client in toothbrush techniques for the pet. The client should approach toothbrush training with the same attitude as other forms of training—that is, use lots of praise and lots of patience. The pet first needs to be in an area where it feels confident and comfortable; for small pets, this is often the client's lap. The pet should become familiar with having the muzzle handled. Once at ease with handling, the client should wrap a small cloth, strip of nylon hose, or strip of gauze around the index finger. The pet should have only one or two teeth wiped during early training sessions. The client can gradually begin to introduce the toothbrush as both client and pet become familiar with the routine.

A soft-bristled toothbrush matching the pet's mouth size should be dispersed or recommended. Different suggestions could be made to the client to aid in remembering to brush the pet's teeth and making brushing a positive experience. The locations suggested for brushing might limit, to a certain extent, other recommendations. For instance, if the pet is most comfortable in the owner's lap, it might be suggested that the owner keep the pet's toothbrush next to a favorite chair and that it be used dry and rinsed later. This activity often coordinates well with watching a specific daily television program. Other locations might include the bathroom just before bedtime or the kitchen after dishes are done. The client will be more likely to remember to brush the pet's teeth if brushing can become behavior-associated—that is, a habit.

Special doggie toothpastes are available (DVM* and Doggy-Dent*) and may appeal to some clients and their pets. These toothpastes are flavored and may indeed affect the pet's reaction to having the teeth brushed. Human toothpastes were used three times daily in toothpaste tests in Beagle colonies without adverse effects.[6] It should be remembered, however, that toothpastes, canine and human, contain some sodium, and their use should be restricted in cardiac patients. Sodium chloride and sodium bicarbonate are not recommended as dentifrices for the same reason.

There are currently being produced or nearing FDA approval several plaque-inhibiting agents. Some are incorporated in a dentifrice (Dentagard†), whereas others will be in a gel form (Biotene‡). Fluoride is a component of many human toothpastes and is also available in gel. A solution of 0.2 per cent chlorhexadine digluconate has been approved in Europe as an effective supragingival plaque-inhibitor. It is not yet available in the United States. This solution is extremely bitter, and human patients sometimes complain that taste sensation is altered adversely.[8] These facts should be taken into consideration before chlorhexadine is dispensed. There may be justification in recommending these products to pet owners for use in wiping on the teeth, brushing on the teeth, or simply flushing the mouth.

There will be clients and pets who will not or cannot participate in dental home care. Client education in toothbrushing is necessary in these cases to make the client aware that because of the *lack* of home care, more frequent dental prophylaxes may be essential for the pet's dentition and general health.

Adjuncts to dental care for the pet include the use of dry food versus canned and the use of dental exercisers. Hard treats and hard rubber chew toys serve to exercise the periodontal ligaments and preserve their function.

RESCHEDULING

The dental patient should be re-evaluated on an individual basis depending on its dental health. The puppy or kitten should be checked for bite problems at each visit and scheduled at 7 to 9 months of age to examine the mouth for retained deciduous teeth. Pets should be evaluated yearly for a dental prophylaxis. Pets with periodontal disease should be scheduled as often as needed to

---

*DVM Doggy Dent, San Mateo, California.
†Colgate-Palmolive, Norwood, Massachusetts.
‡Henry Schein, Inc., Port Washington, New York.

maintain their oral health. This may be as frequent as 1 to 3 months in the severely affected pet, 3 to 6 months for moderate disease, and yearly for those with minimal change. If home care is being maintained at an acceptable level, the frequency of repeat dental prophylaxes can be decreased.

SUMMARY

Success in veterinary dentistry lies in good home care and regular, thorough dental prophylaxis. The removal of supragingival and subgingival calculus must be accomplished before periodontal disease can be controlled. When gingival sulcus depths exceed 4 or 5 mm, the gingivae must be excised or reflected to allow proper treatment of the pocket area. Antibiotic therapy should be instituted in the extensively involved veterinary dental patient.

REFERENCES

1. Dietrich, U. B.: Dental care: Prophylaxis and therapy. Canine Pract., 3:44–53, 1976.
2. Freed, H., and Charles, A. H.: Review of periodontal surgery. Continuing Education Series. Portland, Oregon Health Sciences University, 1984.
3. Grant, D., Stern, I., and Everett, F.: Orban's Periodontics. St. Louis, C. V. Mosby Co., 1968.
4. Grove, T. K.: Periodontal disease. Compend. Contin. Ed. Pract. Vet., 4(7):564, 1982.
5. Grove, T. K.: Periodontal disease. In Harvey, C. E. (ed.): Veterinary Dentistry. Philadelphia, W. B. Saunders Co., 1985.
6. Johnson, G.: Personal communication. Cincinnati, Ohio, Proctor & Gambel Research Division, 1984.
7. Lane, J. G.: Small animal dentistry. J. Small Anim. Pract., 2(3): 1981.
8. Lindhe, J.: Textbook of Clinical Periodontology. Edition 1. Philadelphia, W. B. Saunders Co., 1983.
9. Musselman, E. E.: Bacterial endocarditis. III. Veterinary Professional Topics. University of Illinois, College of Veterinary Medicine, Volume 6, Number 2, 1981.
10. Parkes, R. B., and Kolstad, R. A.: Effects of sterilization on periodontal instruments. J. Periodont., 53:434–436, 1982.
11. Pattison, A. M., and Behrens, J.: Dental Hygiene: The Detection and Removal of Calculus. Reston, Virginia, Reston Publishing Co., 1973.
12. Ross, D. L.: The oral cavity. In Kirk, R. W. (ed.): Current Veterinary Therapy VII. Philadelphia, W. B. Saunders Co., 1977.
13. Schluger, S., Yuodelis, R. A., and Page, R. C.: Periodontal Disease. Philadelphia, Lea & Febiger, 1977.
14. Short, T.: Smarten Up, Sharpen Up. Chicago, Hu-Friedy, Inc., 1982.
15. Tholen, M.: Concepts of Veterinary Dentistry. Edwardsville, Kansas, Veterinary Medicine Publishing Co., 1983.
16. Williams, C. A.: The use of rotary ultrasonic scalers in small animal veterinary dentistry. Am. Vet. Dent. Newsletter, 2(2):2, 1985.

Orchard Animal Clinic
110 North Orchard Street
Boise, Idaho 83706

Feline Dental Disease

Patricia Frost, D.V.M.,* and Charles A. Williams, D.V.M.†

Feline dental disease is frequently seen in veterinary medicine. Until recently, little has been written or studied on specific feline dental problems such as the chronic gingivitis/stomatitis syndrome and the subgingival resorptive lesions or "neck lesions" that are frequently seen. As the cat has become more popular and the purebred cat important as a showing and breeding animal, owners are becoming more interested in the health care of their animals, including oral health. A survey was taken in 1985 by the American Veterinary Dental Society (AVDS) of its members and members of the American Association of Feline Practitioners to establish a baseline of what is being seen and done in practice with feline dental diseases. Results from this survey are given throughout the article. In this article, we hope to provide a report of feline diseases and their current treatment.

DENTITION, ANATOMY, AND OCCLUSION

The feline mouth is designed for grasping, tearing, and shearing, as is the canine mouth, but with a much shorter muzzle. Therefore, the cat has fewer teeth and a much smaller buccal cavity than the dog. The permanent dentition in the cat is made up of 30 teeth with the dental formula as follows:[24]

$$I - \frac{3}{3} \quad C - \frac{1}{1} \quad P - \frac{3}{2} \quad M - \frac{1}{1}$$

---
*Veterinary Dental Services, Roosevelt Roads Naval Station, Ceiba, Puerto Rico
†Director, Blue Cross Animal Hospital, Fairfax, Virginia

The primary (deciduous) teeth start erupting during the second or third week of age and eruption is complete by the fourth week, with a dentition of 26 teeth. The dental formula for a kitten is as follows:[24]

$$I - \frac{3}{3} C - \frac{1}{1} P - \frac{3}{2}$$

The eruption of the permanent teeth is variable but usually starts with the central incisors at 3 to 4 months. The remaining incisors follow shortly, and the permanent canine appears at 4 to 5 months. The lower molar is one of the first caudal teeth to erupt along with the upper P1. The eruption process is usually complete with the crowns fully exposed by 6 months of age.[2]

The anatomy of the teeth, with prominent pointed crowns, is similar to a dog's. The incisors are very small with long roots. They have three cusps, with the central cusp being slightly higher than the others. The canine teeth have a slightly curved, sharply pointed crown with a prominent vertical groove in the lateral surface of the upper canines. The upper first premolar is a small, single-rooted tooth. The second upper premolar, lower first premolar, and second lower premolar are similar teeth with a central cusp taller than the smaller basal cusps and two roots of similar size and length. The third upper premolar has three roots and a large central cusp. The two smaller rostral roots lie side by side, with the large caudal root situated rostrocaudal. The upper molar is very small and is situated transversely. It has two roots and the crown has a grinding surface. The lower molar is large with two prominent cusps. It has two roots, with the rostral root being quite large and the caudal root significantly smaller. The third upper premolar and the lower molar are the carnassial teeth[24] (Fig. 1).

The structure of the feline tooth is similar to the dog's. There is a crown, a neck, which is more prominent in the premolars and molars, and a root. The crown is made up of enamel on the outer surface, with dentin underlying the enamel and making up the majority of the root. The pulp cavity lies in the center of the tooth and consists of the blood vessels, nerves, and connective tissue of the tooth. The root is held in place by periodontal ligament fibers embedded in the cementum that covers the root dentin and attached to the alveolar bone of the tooth socket. The gingival tissue surrounding the teeth is tightly adherent to the tooth at the cementoenamel junction and normally does not have a sulcus depth greater than 1 to 2 mm.

The cat has fewer problems with dentition compared with the dog, but variations do occur. Missing teeth are rare in young animals

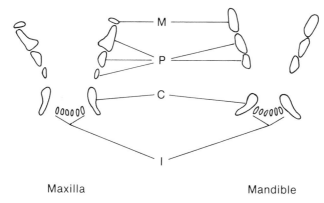

Figure 1. Schematic representation of teeth in upper and lower jaws. *I* = incisor. *C* = canine. *P* = premolar. *M* = molar.

and are usually due to early loss secondary to periodontal disease in older animals. Incisors are the first to be lost and may be missing as early as 2 years of age. A case of total anodontia has been reported in a male domestic shorthair.[10] The animal was unable to breed, possibly owing to its inability to grab the queen's neck skin during mating.

Extra teeth are more frequently seen, with retained primary canine teeth being the most common. In the AVDS survey, approximately 25 per cent of the respondents see extra teeth as frequently as one or more times a month. Retained primary teeth should be removed when they are seen to prevent early periodontal disease due to the collection of food, hair, and calculus between the teeth and to prevent a malocclusion. Care should be taken to remove the entire primary canine tooth root. Making a small incision laterally in the gingiva over the root and careful manipulation with a small root elevator will increase the success of complete removal of the root. The incision can be left to heal by second intention or a few interrupted sutures with absorbable suture can be placed. Retained root tips may act as a foreign body and create an abscess or fistula.

Occlusion variations are infrequently seen in the cat. In the AVDS survey, fewer than 20 per cent of the respondents reported seeing malocclusions once a month or more. The most common malocclusion seen is protruding canines, where the lower canines are angled rostrally to varying degrees. This causes interference with the soft tissues of the lip and creates an uncosmetic appearance. These exposed canines are more susceptible to trauma and periodontal disease. Options for these teeth are extraction, orthodontic manipulation, or shortening the crown tip to prevent soft-tissue injury.

Other malocclusions that are seen are (1) brachygnathism, where

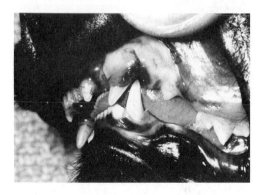

Figure 2. Brachygnathic malocclusion in a young cat, causing
soft-tissue trauma.

the mandible is shorter than the maxilla; (2) wry mouth, where one side of either the mandible or the maxilla has grown longer than the other, creating a crooked jaw appearance and malalignment of the teeth; (3) prognathism, with the mandible being longer than the maxilla; and (4) anterior crossbite, where one or more of the upper incisors are just behind the lower incisors with the rest of the occlusion being normal. The problems caused by these malocclusions will vary with the severity of the disruption of the normal occlusal pattern. Normally, the upper incisors come just in front of the lower incisors in a "scissor" bite. The canines interdigitate with each other, with the mandibular canine coming up between the upper canine and the lateral incisor forming a dental interlock, and come to the outside of the opposite jaw. There is little contact between premolars and molars other than the shearing action of the carnassial teeth and the grinding surface of the upper molar. When teeth are out of alignment, they may abnormally contact each other or soft tissues causing excessive wear or trauma or predisposing the animal to periodontal disease (Fig. 2). Treatment should be directed toward removing these abnormal contact points by extracting offending teeth, shortening crowns with endodontic treatment or, in some cases, with orthodontic manipulations. Purebred cats—the Persian, in particular, with its brachycephalic head type—are more likely to show these malocclusions, possibly owing to the lack of the proper dental interlock between the canines and upper lateral incisor allowing variations in the jaw length.

PERIODONTAL DISEASE

Periodontal disease is the most common dental disease in cats. In the AVDS survey, nearly 90 per cent of the veterinarians responding reported seeing two or more cases a week with dental calculus and periodontal disease. Unfortunately, there have been few studies done to evaluate the incidence and pathogenesis of periodontal disease in cats. In a 1982 European study of 200 healthy cats that were anesthetized and examined orally for dental disease, 57.5 per cent were found to have mild to severe gingivitis/periodontitis.[20] In this study, purebred cats were found to have a higher incidence of dental calculus than the European shorthair, with the Siamese being the most affected.

The pathogenesis of periodontal disease in cats appears to start out similar to that in dogs, with the accumulation of plaque on the tooth surface, which initiates an inflammatory response in the gingival sulcus. The premolars and molars are the first teeth to show this accumulation. This plaque becomes mineralized to form calculus, and the inflammatory process in the gingival sulcus continues. The appearance of calculus with marginal gingivitis can be seen as early as 2 years of age. The calculus accumulation is greatest on the maxillary premolars and molar and on the buccal versus lingual surface.[17] The bacterial populations that are involved in the production of plaque and the ongoing inflammatory process in the gingival sulcus have not been thoroughly studied. Oral bacteria that have been isolated in the cat are *Pasteurella multocida*, *Staphylococcus albus*, various streptococci species, and *Neisseiria*.[17] The exact role of these bacteria in the pathogenesis of feline periodontal disease has not been determined.

The accumulation of plaque and calculus leads to a marginal gingivitis with increased vascular proliferation of the gingival papillae. Inflammatory infiltrates made up of mostly lymphocytes and plasma cells are seen in the gingival tissue. With increased cellular infiltrations there is apical migration of the crevicular epithelium and formation of the periodontal pocket. The lining of the pocket becomes eroded with areas of sloughed epithelium. As the periodontal ligament is destroyed by the inflammatory process, the periodontal pocket deepens and there is alveolar bone resorption. There can be both horizontal and vertical bone loss. There is a greater degree of alveolar bone resorption seen around the canines and incisors even though little plaque and calculus may be noted. As the pocket deepens, there is accumulation of pus and debris and eventual loss of the tooth. Early tooth loss is the result of progressive periodontitis, and the incisors and premolars are the first to go. Of the 200 cats in the European study, 125 cats were missing 811 teeth.[20] Tooth loss increases with age, and upper teeth are lost more frequently than lower teeth.

Cats are less apt to develop the proliferative or hyperplastic gingiva than are dogs, although gingival proliferation has been studied in cats given diphenylhydantoin sodium (Dilantin) as a model for humans.[11]

A major difference between the progression of periodontal disease in cats and dogs is the finding of defects at the cementoenamel junction and beyond in cats. These defects are thought to be due to inflammatory resorption caused by periodontal inflammation.[17] These defects have been termed "neck lesions" and may be found in 25 per cent of the teeth affected by periodontal disease.[17] These resorptive lesions can be quite extensive and lead to early root fracture with subsequent tooth loss, leaving a retained root tip in the alveolar bone. Fistula formation with epithelial proliferation and subepithelial inflammatory infiltrates and cysts can be seen with these retained roots.[17]

Factors leading to periodontal disease in cats have not been fully determined. The feeding of soft and canned, commercially prepared foods has been shown to increase the amount of plaque and calculus formation over the feeding of dry food.[25] The 1982 European study, however, did not find a similar correlation to diet and housing with the incidence of periodontal disease and accumulations of calculus. The feeding of raw liver was noted to increase the number of resorptive lesions found, although the number of cats on this diet was small.[20]

The action of salivary enzymes is felt to be contributory to calculus production in dogs owing to the accumulation of greater amounts of calculus found opposite salivary gland openings in the mouth. Cats that had their parotid, submaxillary, and sublingual glands removed formed the same amount of calculus as the control cats fed the same diet.[18]

CLINICAL SIGNS

Cats with periodontal disease may show variable clinical signs depending upon the severity of the disease. Mild cases may show moderate amounts of calculus formation and a marginal gingivitis with increased bleeding on probing. There may be a slight halitosis noted by the owner, but the cat is usually not showing signs of discomfort. Siamese cats, however, will often have a more severe gingivitis in relation to the amount of calculus present.

As the periodontitis progresses, there is an increased accumulation of calculus, gingival swelling, pocket formation of 3 to 4 mm, and teeth that are loose. These animals may show a reluctance to eat hard foods, there is a prominent halitosis, and a variable amount of gingival bleeding (Fig. 3).

Severe periodontal disease presents with massive amounts of

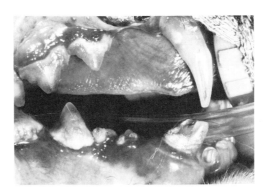

Figure 3. Cat with moderate calculus accumulation, gingivitis, gingival recession around maxillary canine tooth, and fractured lower canine tooth.

calculus with gingival recession and exposed tooth roots. The gingiva is swollen and hyperemic; pus and debris can be found around loose teeth; and some teeth may be missing. These cats may be anorectic, less active, paw at the mouth, and show general discomfort around the mouth. They may be difficult to examine orally unless sedated (Fig. 4).

TREATMENT

Prevention is the best treatment, and all cats would benefit from routine dental prophylaxis to remove the accumulated plaque and calculus and treat the gingivitis before it progresses to irreversible periodontitis. Even older cats with more severe forms of periodontal disease will benefit from extraction of loose and painful teeth and the elimination of the source of infection in their mouth.

The treatment of periodontal disease in cats consists of removal of dental calculus and plaque, subgingival scaling and curettage,

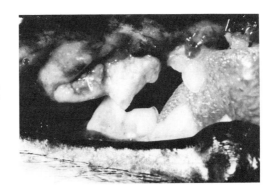

Figure 4. Cat with severe periodontal disease of maxillary premolars and molars.

examination for periodontal pockets, and subgingival resorptive lesions of the roots, along with extracting hopeless teeth. Scaling can be done very effectively using hand scalers in the cat because of the smaller size and number of teeth. The premolars and molars will be the teeth to concentrate on because they will have the greatest calculus accumulation. The use of an ultrasonic scaler is effective if care is taken not to injure the gingiva. The cat must have an endotracheal tube in place with the cuff inflated, even if an injectable anesthetic is used, to prevent inhalation of the aerosol produced. The vertical groove on the lateral surface on the canine tooth will accumulate plaque and calculus and should be cleaned thoroughly. An eight-sided, pointed, finishing bur in a dental handpiece is very effective for this.

Special attention should be given to the subgingival area. The removal of subgingival calculus with very fine scalers or curettes will prevent undue trauma to the friable gingiva that is freqently seen in cats with marginal gingivitis. If a high-speed dental handpiece is available, the use of a Roto Pro bur (rotary ultrasonic scaler) is very useful in cats, as the tip is very fine and can be used for removal of subgingival calculus and root planing in pockets up to 3 to 4 mm deep without injuring the gingiva. Root planing smoothes the root surface and allows for reattachment of healthy gum tissue. All subgingival areas should be explored for subgingival resorptive lesions. (Treatment of these lesions is discussed later in this article.)

Tooth mobility should be checked using a finger or the blunt end of a single-end instrument. Any teeth that are loose or that have greater than 50 per cent of the root or the bifurcation exposed should be extracted. Extracting teeth in cats must be done with care, as the roots are easily fractured. Careful use of a fine-tipped root elevator to break down the periodontal ligament fibers and splitting of all multirooted teeth will make complete extractions easier. A no. 65 extraction forcep that has small, pointed tips that come together is useful for removing the loosened tooth. Retained root tips should be removed by flushing out the alveolar socket to visualize the shiny white tip and using an apical elevator or a root tip pick to work the fragment out of the socket. A high-speed dental handpiece can be used to drill out the retained fragments if available.

Gingivectomy and gingival flap techniques are effective in cats with hyperplastic gingiva and deep pockets. Polishing after scaling is necessary to provide a smooth enamel surface and remove any microscopic etches made by the instruments to slow down the accumulation of future plaque and calculus. A thorough final flushing will remove any polishing paste and debris from the subgingival area, leaving the mouth clean and the cat presentable for discharge after recovery from the anesthetic.

Home care for cats is important for both prevention and control of periodontal disease. It includes attention to diet and brushing or rubbing the teeth to remove the daily accumulation of plaque. Many clients are not able or willing to go to this effort, and many cats are less than willing to have it done; therefore, recommendations for more frequent routine dental prophylaxis should be made to maintain healthier teeth and detect problems before they become advanced. In the AVDS survey, 65 per cent of the respondents said that less than 20 per cent of their feline clients were on a routine dental care program. A few respondents who reported a higher percentage mentioned that they routinely "chipped off" the calculus on the caudal teeth when cats were presented for annual vaccinations. Ninety-three per cent of the survey respondents reported fewer than 20 per cent of their clients following a home oral hygiene program with their cats. Several noted that the owners were willing but the cats were not. Most cats, with some training and lots of patience, can be taught to allow their teeth to be brushed or rubbed with gauze. The benefits of this in preventing calculus build-up were reported by Richardson, showing that cats that had their teeth brushed daily or two times per week had 95 per cent less calculus formation than the controls. Even cats that had their teeth brushed once a week had a 76 per cent reduction in calculus formation.[18] Painting the gums with hydrogen peroxide, glyoxide, or chlorhexidine gel may also be beneficial and less distressing to the cat than brushing.

SUBGINGIVAL RESORPTIVE LESIONS

These lesions were first thought to be carious lesions,[13, 27] but were later described as a progressive, subgingival, osteoclastic resorption.[19] They are apparently a recent development in the cat, as Colyer did not describe these lesions in his examination of 341 cat skulls.[5] These defects were termed "neck lesions" because they appear at the cementoenamel junction and are often not identified without subgingival exploration. The premolars and molars are the most likely teeth to be affected, but these lesions have been found in the canine teeth and incisors. These lesions were found on the buccal surface in 83 per cent of the teeth affected in one study,[21] but were described as being located on 34.4 per cent of the facial (buccal) surface of premolars and molars and 29 per cent of the oral (lingual) surface of these teeth in another.[17] These defects are often covered with calculus and may not be noted until the calculus is removed. The lesions may also be covered by hyperplastic gingiva and filled with granulation tissue. The cats are often reluctant to eat

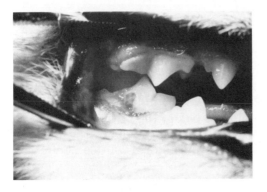

Figure 5. Subgingival resorptive lesion in mandibular molar of a young cat. Note the minimal calculus accumulation on the teeth and absence of periodontal disease.

hard food. When some lesions are probed when the cat is under anesthesia, they are quite painful, as evidenced by a jaw twitch.

Affected cats are generally middle-aged, but these lesions have been found in cats as young as 2 years of age. There appears to be no sex predisposition. Purebred cats were the most susceptible, with the Siamese and Persian having the most lesions in the 1982 European study.[20] Cats may have multiple teeth affected with different stages of the lesion.

As these lesions progress, they increase in size. Defects in their early stages can be seen in calculus-free teeth (Fig. 5). These early defects are amenable to restoration with amalgam or composite resin (technique described later in this article). As the lesion progresses and enlarges, it may involve one or both roots and may go all the way through the root. When the lesion is explored with a probe, the dentin is hard and not softened as in a typical carious lesion. Histologically, the lesion is described as being a half moon depression of varying depth, located at the cementoenamel junction.[17, 21] The surrounding dentin is normal and there is no inflammatory reaction observed in the pulp tissue. The depression is lined with osteoclasts. Repair attempts with an osteodentin-like material are seen in some lesions.

The etiology of these resorptive lesions has not been completely determined. Although the process resembles inflammatory resorption as opposed to surface or replacement absorption, very early lesions are covered by apparently normal gingiva.[17] Commercial diets don't seem to be a factor, because in 14 wild cat skulls studied from the Natural History Museum of Bern, Switzerland, one neck lesion was described. Out of 244 skulls of "gone wild" cats that were studied from the museum, 58 had one or more neck lesion.[19] Feeding of raw liver is associated with an increased number of lesions.[19, 20]

There may be a significant correlation between chronic recurrent gingivitis/stomatitis cases and the finding of subgingival lesions. In

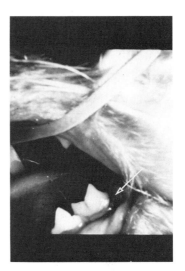

Figure 6. Amalgam restoration of a subgingival resorptive lesion in mandibular molar.

the AVDS survey, 34 per cent of respondents replied that the syndrome was frequently associated with these lesions. More studies are needed to further define the incidence of "neck lesions" and determine their relationship to periodontal disease and gingivitis and the association with raw liver diets.

TREATMENT

Treatment is usually extraction of the involved tooth, making sure that any root tips remaining in the alveolar socket are removed. When resorptive lesions are seen at an early stage before they create a root fracture or enter the pulp, the tooth can be preserved by doing a restorative procedure and filling the defect (Fig. 6). To get the best exposure to drill out the defect and prepare it for filling, a gingival flap is necessary. Cautery or hemostatic agents can be used to reduce the bleeding and keep the area visible. The lesion is prepared for the filling material using a small no. 1 or 2 round bur or a no. 34 or 35 inverted cone bur to smooth the edges of the lesion, remove any discolored dentin, and make an undercut to retain the filling material. Owing to the small size, it is often difficult to make the necessary undercut to retain an amalgam filling, and the composite resin materials that bond to dentin may be preferable. The gingival flap is sutured in place with absorbable suture. The success rate is excellent initially, as the cats are pain free and they eat and feel better. Without consistent oral hygiene at home, the possibility of finding new lesions with time is good and the owner

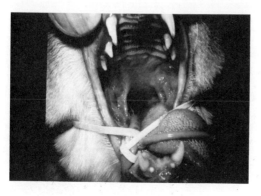

Figure 7. Chronic gingivitis/
stomatitis in 6-month-old Siamese.

should be encouraged to initiate an oral hygiene program at home
for their pet to prevent new lesions from appearing.

GINGIVITIS/ STOMATITIS

Chronic gingivitis/stomatitis is the second most frequently seen
dental disease in cats. Thirty-nine per cent of the AVDS survey
respondents reported seeing cases two or more times per week, with
another 23 per cent seeing cases at least once a week. This disease
is seen in all breeds, but certain breeds are more frequently
associated with this problem. Siamese are the most commonly
mentioned, with Abyssinians, Persians, Himalayans, and Burmese
being listed in the AVDS survey. This disease syndrome can affect
animals of all ages. Young cats less than 2 years old generally start
out with a persistent marginal gingivitis that may progress with age
to a more generalized gingivitis/stomatitis.

Cats may present with gingival hyperemia, swelling, ulceration,
and proliferation in the premolar and molar area. In some cases, this
proliferation may extend to the glossopalatine arches, pharynx, and
hard palate (Fig. 7). Ulcerations of the tongue may be noted. There
may be concurrent periodontal disease with gingival recession and
loss of teeth. Excessive salivation, halitosis, and decreased appetite
or pain on eating hard food are often noted by the owner. These
cases can be very frustrating for the owner and the clinician. In the
AVDS survey, there were variable results as to the effectiveness of
different types of therapy. There were many types of individual
therapy regimens reported. In order to have a better understanding
of this disease syndrome, its possible causes and treatments are
outlined.

The most common cause of gingivitis is periodontal disease.
This disease may be more severe in cats with diabetes mellitus or

hypothyroidism.[4] Cats that are uremic secondary to chronic renal disease may also have oral ulcerations with an aggravation of concurrent periodontal disease.

Feline leukemia has been associated with cats presenting with ulcerative gingivitis/stomatitis.[1, 7] It is felt that the immunosuppressive effect of the virus is responsible. This association is not consistent, as many cats with severe, chronic gingivitis/stomatitis are negative on the FeLV immunofluorescence test. Only 21 per cent of the veterinarians responding on the AVDS survey felt that cats with this syndrome were often found to be FeLV-positive.

The association of other viruses has been found with ulcerative lesions of the mouth and tongue. Both the feline rhinotracheitis virus and feline calicivirus (picorna virus) have been associated with oral lesions, with or without concurrent respiratory involvement.[4, 15] It is not possible to differentiate between the two diseases from the clinical signs or distribution of the ulceration. Calicivirus has been isolated from the gingival tissues of cats with chronic gingivitis secondary to periodontal disease.[26]

Many cases of ulcerative gingivitis/stomatitis in cats have been described as trenchmouth or Vincent's stomatitis.[16] These cases will have calculus accumulation with inflamed, swollen, and ulcerated necrotic mucous membranes. There may be severe gingival recession, and the mouth is extremely painful. An association of this disease with the presence of spirochetes and fusiform bacilli has led to this diagnosis. These bacteria are present in animals' normal mouths but may be present in increased numbers in cats that are showing evidence of severe gingivitis with oral discomfort or acute pain.[8]

The association of chronic gingivitis cases with the presence of subgingival resorptive lesions is unclear. Nearly 63 per cent of the veterinarians answering the AVDS survey felt that these "neck lesions" were at least occasionally associated with chronic gingivitis, with 34 per cent reporting that they *often* find subgingival resorptive lesions. Whether the neck lesions are primary or develop secondary to the gingival disease and then exacerbate the problem has not been determined. Extraction of these teeth is necessary; removal of any retained root tips will assist treatment. It may be necessary to radiograph persistent cases with missing teeth to rule out the presence of retained root tips that are perpetuating the disease.

Pemphigus and toxic epidermal necrolysis have been reported in the cat.[3, 14, 23] These diseases are uncommon and will generally have other mucocutaneous or skin lesions present associated with the disease. Eosinophilic granuloma complex can also resemble some cases of chronic gingivitis. Biopsy specimens of the affected areas are generally diagnostic for these diseases.

A specific form of chronic gingivitis/stomatitis has been described as plasma cell gingivitis-pharyngitis.[12] There are character-
istically raised proliferative lesions that have a cobblestone or rasp-
berry-like appearance, affecting the glossopalatine arches and
extending to the hard and soft palate and gingiva around the
premolars and molars. These animals usually present with hyper-
salivation, halitosis, and dysphagia. Biopsy specimens reveal sheets
of plasma cells as a submucosal cellular infiltrate. There is ulceration
and proliferation of the mucosa. Findings of a polyclonal gammopathy
along with the plasmacytic infiltrate have led to a suggestion that
this disease syndrome is immune-related. There is the possibility of
a sensitivity to the bacterial population associated with dental plaque.
There may be temporary remission with antibiotics and anti-inflammatory agents and intensive oral hygiene to reduce the bacterial
population, but recurrence is common with discontinuation of therapy. The most successful therapy for these cases is total extraction
of the caudal teeth.

Other causes of gingivitis/stomatitis that must be ruled out are
external trauma, poisoning, nutrition (protein-deficient diets), and
neoplastic diseases.

TREATMENT

Treatment should be as specific as possible. Diagnostic tests to
rule out kidney disease, diabetes mellitus, feline leukemia virus, and
hypothyroidism should be done to eliminate or confirm the involvement of these diseases. Swabs for identification of spirochetes,
fusiform bacteria, and virus isolation may be helpful.

Biopsy specimens from representative lesions are helpful to
identify autoimmune diseases, eosinophilic granuloma complex, neoplastic disease, and plasmacytic gingivitis/stomatitis. A histologic
result of chronic inflammation or granuloma is frequently the case,
and specific treatment is not obvious.

Cats that are presented for the first time with a mild form of
gingivitis/stomatitis should have a thorough dental prophylaxis, with
particular attention given to the subgingival area to remove all
subgingival plaque and calculus and detect any subgingival resorptive
lesions. Loose, abscessed, and hopeless teeth should be extracted.
A dental prophylaxis may be necessary every 3 to 4 months to keep
these cats asymptomatic. Response to the AVDS survey showed that
56 per cent of the veterinarians felt that multiple teeth cleanings
and particularly tooth extractions were often successful, and another
31 per cent felt these procedures were occasionally successful in
resolving these cases.

Home care is an important follow-up to the dental prophylaxis to help remove the daily accumulation of plaque that may be a complicating factor in these cases. Instruction on the use of a small toothbrush or use of gauze over a finger to clean the teeth daily or at least several times a week can be beneficial in reducing the severity of the disease and the frequency of recurrences. Two per cent potassium permanganate or 0.2 per cent chlorhexidine solutions have been recommended to reduce the bacterial population in the mouth and can be used as mouthwashes, painted on the teeth and gingiva, or as a dentrifice.[4, 15, 16]

ANTIMICROBIAL THERAPY

Antibiotics should be used as an adjunct to other therapy, because bacteria are rarely a primary cause of gingivitis/stomatitis; however, they do play a role as a secondary problem. Generally, broad-spectrum antibiotics such as the synthetic penicillins, tetracycline, trimethoprim plus sulfamethoxazole, lincocin, and cephalosporins have been mentioned as being beneficial.[4, 15] Therapy should be continued for at least 21 days and, in some cases, treatment may need to be repeated. Long-term antibiotic therapy runs the risk of fungal overgrowth with organisms such as *Candida* and should be avoided. Topical as well as systemic therapy may be needed. Anaerobic bacteria can be controlled with metronidazole at 30 to 50 mg per kg once a day[4, 8, 15] and may be helpful in cases with high numbers of spirochetes and fusiform bacteria.

ANTI-INFLAMMATORY THERAPY

Glucocorticoids should be used cautiously in cases of gingivitis/stomatitis. When used as an immunosuppressive agent in cases of autoimmune disease, they should be used at an appropriate dose. Prednisolone or prednisone at a dose of 2 to 5 mg per kg per day is immunosuppressive. An initial dose of 1 mg per kg twice a day often results in clinical improvement in those cases that are going to respond. After there is a response to the initial dose at 2 mg per kg per day, the dose should be gradually reduced until alternate-day therapy is reached.[4] Some cases of gingivitis/stomatitis will be steroid-responsive even though there is not confirmation of an immunologic etiology. Plasmacytic gingivitis is one example. Glucocorticoids should not be used in cats that are already immunosuppressed secondary to feline leukemia. Treatment of autoimmune disease may also necessitate the use of cytotoxic drugs such as

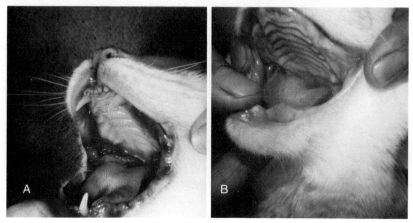

Figure 8. Plasmacytic stomatitis. *A*, After extraction of premolars and molars. *B*, The same cat 1 month after extraction of remaining teeth.

cyclophosphamide and azothioprine. They should be used at recommended doses and one should note their side effects.

Other drugs such as megestrol acetate (Ovaban) and levamisole have been used with varying success. Ovaban is thought to be beneficial for its anti-inflammatory properties. It is also used in the treatment of the eosinophilic granuloma complex. Levamisole is thought to have immunostimulating properties and may be helpful in some cases. The dosage is 2 to 5 mg per kg three times a week. Side effects have been reported with levamisole including nausea, diarrhea, depression, behavioral changes, and central nervous system signs.[4]

In many cases, the most successful treatment is removal of the caudal teeth. This would appear to be a drastic alternative, but the cats that are treated this way generally resolve the severe inflammatory response and they are then able to eat comfortably. In some severe cases, all the teeth have been removed before there was alleviation of the symptoms (Fig. 8). Care should be taken not to leave any broken root tips that would allow the disease condition to persist.

Other treatments that have been reported are the use of gold salts injections (Solganol, 1 mg per week for 8 weeks, then once a month), multiple vitamins, vitamins B, C, and E, zinc, and NaFl added to drinking water. The cat may need to be fed soft food during treatment until the gingiva becomes less painful. Hard food should be offered to provide chewing exercise and some degree of plaque removal.

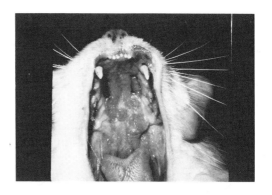

Figure 9. Eosinophilic granuloma lesions on upper lip and hard
palate.

EOSINOPHILIC GRANULOMA COMPLEX

Oral lesions are common in cats with eosinophilic granuloma complex. It has been described in three forms: eosinophilic ulcer, linear granuloma, and eosinophilic plaque.[22] Oral lesions are most commonly seen with the first two forms of the disease and may appear as nodules, plaques, or as a proliferative ulcerated tissue anywhere in the mouth (Fig. 9).[4] The cats exhibit excessive salivation and have difficulty eating owing to the painful lesions in their mouths. Lesions may be present on other parts of the body, and a biopsy is recommended to differentiate them from squamous cell carcinoma when therapy fails to resolve the lesions. Treatment consists of corticosteroids administered systemically, intralesionally, or both. An intralesional injection of 3 mg of triamcinolone can be given weekly in solitary lesions until the lesion has healed. Oral predni-solone at a dose of 1 to 2 mg per kg twice a day has been recommended if the cat will take oral medication. Subcutaneous injections of 20 mg of methylprednisolone acetate per cat are also effective when given every 2 weeks until the lesion has healed. A month or more of therapy may be required for healing to be complete, and treatment should not be discontinued until this time.[4]

If therapy with corticosteroids is unsuccessful, progestational compounds such as megestrol acetate have been used. Recom-mended dosage is 2.5 to 5.0 mg every other day. This dosage should be continued until the lesion has healed.[4] Numerous side effects have been seen with these drugs, and careful monitoring of the cat during treatment should be maintained.

If adequate dosages are used for sufficient duration, most animals will have successful treatment. The recurrence rate is high in those animals that fail to respond to glucocorticoids or that have had a previous lesion that did respond to therapy. The prognosis is poor

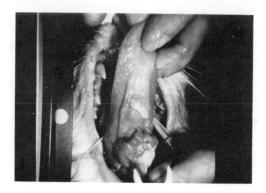

Figure 10. Squamous cell carcinoma at base of tongue.

in those cats that fail to respond to either corticosteroid or progestational compound therapy.

ORAL TUMORS

Oral tumors in cats are the fourth most common tumor type
seen.[6] Affected cats are generally over 10 years of age. Malignant
tumors are most frequently seen, with squamous cell carcinoma
being the most common histologic type.[6, 9] Fibrosarcoma follows
with benign neoplasms being rare in the cat. Odontogenic tumors
are rare, but can be seen in young cats. Malignant tumors are locally
invasive, rapidly growing and late to metastasize. They tend to be
more aggressive in the cat than those seen in the dog; therefore,
early diagnosis is paramount. The most common sites of origin are
the tongue (Fig. 10), gingiva, palate, dental alveoli, and buccal and
labial mucosa.[6] Cats may present with halitosis, oral bleeding,
dysphagia, ulceration, abnormal tissue growth, and dental disease.
Gingival squamous cell carcinomas may initially resemble gingivitis
with loosening of the teeth. Oral tumors are important as a differential diagnosis for other oral diseases such as gingivitis and eosinophilic granuloma, particularly in older cats. Intraoral radiography
and biopsy are beneficial to early diagnosis of a neoplastic process
when aggressive gingival lesions are seen.

To be successful, treatment must be initiated early. Local
excision is generally unsuccessful owing to the invasive nature of
these tumors. Hemimandibulectomy and partial maxillectomy may
be more successful in obtaining greater survival times and some
cures. Results of treatment with radiation therapy and chemotherapy
or immunotherapy have been poor.[6]

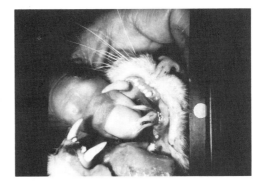

Figure 11. Vertical fracture of left maxillary canine tooth.

FRACTURED TEETH AND ABSCESSED TEETH

Fractured and abscessed teeth are not uncommon in the cat. In the AVDS survey, 60 per cent of the veterinarians reported seeing fractured teeth one or more times a month, with 70 per cent reporting seeing abscessed teeth one or more times a month. Tooth fractures are most frequently seen in males that have access to the outside and are probably caused by fighting, accidents, and falls. The canine tooth is most commonly fractured with the fracture occurring horizontally through the tip or middle of the tooth. Occasionally, vertical fractures occur and are more likely to cause clinical signs (Fig. 11). The outcome of these fractures can be chronic apical periodontitis, pulpitis, necrosis of the pulp, and abscessation of the tooth (Fig. 12). Surprisingly, even with this pathology, many cats are not clinical. Treatment of a fractured tooth will depend on the type of fracture, whether or not the pulp has been exposed, and the desires of the owner. Fractured canines with pulp exposure may be treated endodontically to prevent future pulp necrosis and apical abscess formation and preserve the tooth. Teeth that are already

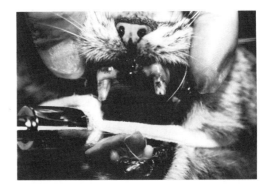

Figure 12. Tom cat with fractured canine teeth and subsequent abscessation.

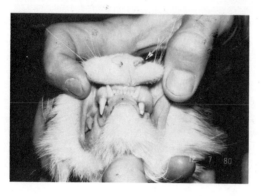

Figure 13. Abscessed maxillary canine tooth with oronasal fistula and nasal discharge.

abscessed, loose, or that have a fracture that extends below the gum line should be extracted.

Abscessed teeth can be caused by fractures that expose the pulp or be secondary to progressive periodontal disease. Canine teeth that are abscessed can lead to subsequent erosion of the nasal bone medial to the tooth root, creating an oronasal fistula. This may present with a nasal discharge, sneezing, and swollen gingiva around the affected tooth (Fig. 13). Facial swelling may also be present. Maxillary sinus involvement is not nearly as common in the cat as it is in the dog. Mandibular teeth that abscess may erode through the mandible and drain ventrally. In all cases, extraction of the tooth and debridement of any necrotic tissue should be performed. Treatment with antibiotics such as penicillin or ampicillin for 4 to 5 days is recommended. Closure of an oronasal fistula can be achieved by creating a mucoperiosteal flap above the defect and pulling it over the opening and suturing the flap to the opposing palatal gingiva.

ENDODONTIC THERAPY

Endodontic therapy in the cat is not frequently done, but two techniques may be used to avoid extraction of otherwise healthy teeth. These are the root canal and the direct pulp capping procedures. A root canal procedure is done to preserve a tooth that has been fractured exposing the pulp. Feline teeth, and particularly the maxillary canine teeth, are apt to undergo early apical resorption when fractured, and a radiograph is helpful to identify these teeth before endodontic treatment is initiated. Another indication of apical resorption is when the endodontic file does not meet resistance at the expected length of the tooth, when it passes through the apex. Teeth with apical resorption are not good candidates for endodontic therapy and should be extracted.

Enlarging the access hole, removing the pulp tissue, and preparing the canal with standard human endodontic files is performed using standard techniques. A calcium hydroxide filling material is used to fill the pulp cavity due to its stimulation of an apical seal by secondary dentin. It can be used alone or with gutta percha points. The access hole can be filled with amalgam or a composite resin. Root canal therapy can be very successful in the cat if done before apical root resorption occurs.

Direct pulp capping can be performed when it is necessary to shorten the crown of a tooth to prevent abnormal occlusion with other teeth or with interference of soft tissues.

ORTHODONTIC PROCEDURES

Fortunately, malocclusion problems are not very common in the cat. For cases that have one or more protruding lower canines, it is possible to return the tooth to a normal position by exerting a caudal force on the tooth. This can be done by placing a small gauge wire in a figure-eight pattern around the two premolars at the tooth neck. The wire is tightened down and a small loop or hook is formed with the twisted end. A ⅛- or ¼-inch orthodontic elastic band is placed from the canine to the wire loop. It will be necessary to bond a small plastic bracket to the canine or secure the elastic with a small amount of composite resin or orthodontic cement. The elastic bands are left in place until the tooth has moved into the desired position. Care must be taken to have the owner clean the area around the wire and canine tooth to remove accumulated plaque and debris to minimize the gingivitis.

Acrylic appliances can be designed to direct displaced canine teeth by designing an incline plane for a palatal appliance in a plaster mold. Cats will usually accept an appliance if it fits properly, but keeping them clean is more difficult, as it is not easy to convince cats to have their mouths cleaned with a water pik.

Many malocclusions in cats are probably hereditary, and correction should not be done just to allow them to be shown. If the malocclusion is causing trauma and discomfort, it is best to require that the animal be neutered if orthodontic manipulations are used to correct the bite. If the malocclusion is due to trauma, a chewing vice, or a developmental defect, orthodontic techniques to correct the occlusion are appropriate.

SUMMARY

Periodontal disease and chronic gingivitis/stomatitis are the most common feline dental diseases. With routine dental care and increased emphasis on home oral hygiene, these diseases can be controlled. Cats can be seen with a number of other dental disorders, and improved treatment methods such as restorations of early subgingival resorptive lesions, endodontic therapy, and orthodontic therapy can be performed successfully. More study and research are necessary about the gingivitis/stomatitis syndrome and subgingival resorptive lesions so that improved prevention and treatment recommendations can be made.

REFERENCES

1. Barrett, R. E., Post, J. E., and Schultz, R. D.: Chronic relapsing stomatitis in a cat associated with feline leukemia virus infection. Feline Pract., 5:34–38, 1975.
2. Berman, E.: The time and pattern of eruption of the permanent teeth of the cat. Lab. Anim. Sci., 24:929–931, 1974.
3. Brown, N. O., and Hurvitz, A. I.: A mucocutaneous disease in a cat resembling human pemphigus. J. Am. Anim. Hosp. Assoc., 15:25–28, 1979.
4. Burrows, C. F., Miller, W. H., and Harvey, C. E.: Oral medicine. In Harvey, C. E. (ed.): Veterinary Dentistry. Philadelphia, W. B. Saunders Co., 1985, pp. 34–58.
5. Colyer, F.: Variations and the Diseases of Teeth of Animals. London, John Bale, Sons and Danielsson. 1936.
6. Cotter, S. M.: Oral pharyngeal neoplasms in the cat. J. Am. Anim. Hosp. Assoc., 17:917–920, 1981.
7. Cotter, S. M., Hardy, W. D., and Essex, M.: Association of feline leukemia virus with lymphosarcoma and other disorders in the cat. J. Am. Vet. Med. Assoc., 166:449–454, 1975.
8. Dean, T. S., Shinn, D. L. S., McFadzean, J. A., et al.: Metronidazole in the treatment of gingivitis. Vet. Rec., 85:449–450, 1969.
9. Dubielzig, R. R.: Proliferative dental and gingival diseases of dogs and cats. J. Am. Anim. Hosp. Assoc., 18:577–584, 1982.
10. Elzay, R. P., and Hughes, R. D.: Anodontia in a cat. J. Am. Vet. Med. Assoc., 154:667–670, 1969.
11. Ishikawa, J., and Glickman, I.: Gingival response to the systemic administration of sodium diphenylhydantoin (Dilatin) in cats. J. Periodontol., 32:149–158, 1961.
12. Johnessee, J. S., and Hurvitz, A. I.: Feline plasma cell gingivitis-pharyngitis. J. Am. Anim. Hosp. Assoc., 19:179–181, 1983.
13. Joshua, J. O.: The Clinical Aspects of Some Diseases of Cats. London, W. Heinemann, 1965, p. 51.
14. Manning, T. O., Scott, D. W., Smith, C. A., et al.: Pemphigus diseases in the feline: Seven case reports and discussion. J. Am. Anim. Hosp. Assoc., 18:433–443, 1982.
15. MacDonald, J. M.: Stomatitis. Vet. Clin. North Am. [Small Anim. Pract.], 13:3, 415–436, 1983.
16. Prescott, C. W.: Some oral lesions in the cat. Aust. Vet. J., 47:41–45, 1971.
17. Reichart, P. A., et al.: Periodontal disease in the domestic cat: A histologic study. J. Periodont. Res., 19:67–75, 1984.
18. Richardson, R.: Dental calculus accumulation in cats. J. Small Anim. Pract., 6(6):475–476, 1965.
19. Schenck, G. W.: Neck lesions in the teeth of cats. Vet. Rec., 99:100, 1976.

20. Von Schlup, D.: Epidemiologische und morphologische Untersuchungen am KatzengebiB I. Mitteilung: Epidemiologische Untersuchungen. Kleinterpraxis, 27:87–94, 1982.
21. Von Schlup, D., and Stich, H.: Epidemiologische und morphologische Untersuchungen am KatzengebiB II. Mitteilung: Morphologische Untersuchungen der "neck lesions." Kleinterpraxis, 27:179–188, 1982.
22. Scott, D. W.: Observations on the eosinophilic granuloma complex in cats. J. Am. Anim. Hosp. Assoc., 11:261–270, 1975.
23. Scott, D. W., Halliwell, R. E. W., and Goldschmidt, M. H.: Toxic epidermal necrolysis in two dogs and a cat. J. Am. Anim. Hosp. Assoc., 15:271–279, 1979.
24. Sisson and Grossman, Anatomy of the Domestic Animals. Edition 5. Philadelphia, W. B. Saunders Co., 1975.
25. Studer, E., and Stapley, R. B.: The role of dry foods in maintaining healthy teeth and gums in the cat. Vet. Med. Small Anim. Clin., 68:1124–1126, 1973.
26. Thompson, R. R., Wilcox, G. E., Clark, W. T., et al.: Association of calicivirus infection with chronic gingivitis and pharyngitis in cats. J. Small Anim. Pract., 25:207–210, 1984.
27. Wilkinson, G. T.: Diseases of the Cat. Oxford, Pergamon Press, 1966, p. 47.

Veterinary Dental Services
Roosevelt Roads Naval Station
Box 3404
FPO Miami, Florida 34051

0195–5616/86 $0.00 + .20

Endodontics

Charles A. Williams, D.V.M.*

The oral examination has long been a part of most veterinary practitioners' check-ups for small animal patients. Hardly a week goes by when the average clinician does not see a fractured tooth, a worn tooth with pulp exposure, a tooth with pupal hemorrhage, or some other cause of pulp death and/or necrosis. Unfortunately, these endodontically diseased teeth are most often overlooked and left to abscess or else they are extracted.[15] An endodontically diseased tooth is not only painful for the pet while it remains untreated, but it is also a source for infection that could affect any part of the body[1, 3, 8] (Fig. 1). Although extraction is a viable solution in some cases, it is often not necessary. Teeth in small animals respond well to endodontic therapy—most often lasting the rest of the pet's life without further problems.[1, 3, 10, 11, 20]

ENDODONTIC THERAPY

Endodontic therapy refers to any procedure that can be employed to treat a tooth with disease of the pulp. For veterinary purposes, pulp therapy might be classified as (1) procedures that are designed to treat and save vital pulp; (2) procedures that retain, but mummify, the pulp; or (3) procedures that remove the pulp altogether.

The process of treating and saving the vital pulp is referred to as pulpotomy with direct pulp capping. Pulpotomy is the removal of the coronal part of the pulp. Direct pulp capping is the placement of medicaments in contact with the remaining vital pulp to induce healing and serve as a thermal buffer between the pulp and the crown restoration.

---

*Director, Blue Cross Animal Hospital, Inc., Fairfax, Virginia

Mummification of the pulp, sometimes referred to as therapeutic pulpotomy, refers to the use of formocreosote or other chemical agents that render the pulp inert, fixed, and incapable of bacterial or autolytic breakdown.[21] The use of this procedure may be indicated due to its ease of performance, but to date, it has not been widely accepted by veterinary dentists and, thus, will not be discussed further in this article.

Pulpectomy, or complete removal of the pulp material, is the most commonly used method of pulp therapy in small animals. This procedure, which is commonly referred to as a "root canal," employs files or reamers to remove all pulp material, disinfectants and cleansing solutions to flush the canal, and inert materials to fill and seal the canal.

In a young animal, the pulp is necessary for tooth growth and development. When a permanent tooth first erupts, it is a shell-like structure—very hard, inorganic enamel covers a relatively thin layer of dentin and a large pulp cavity that contains nerve tissue and blood vessels and is lined with odontoblasts.[6, 25] These odontoblasts produce dentin. As the tooth matures, the dentinal layer becomes thicker and the pulp canal shrinks. Once a tooth has fully matured (by about 18 months of age), it can function well without any pulp at all. In other words, a fully developed tooth is held in place and maintains its integrity from the structures surrounding the root not from its internal parts. Therefore, if the pulp becomes diseased, the pulp can be rendered inert and the tooth kept fully functional by endodontic therapy. If endodontic therapy cannot performed, then the diseased tooth should be extracted.[1, 3, 7, 10, 11, 15, 16, 24]

INDICATIONS FOR ENDODONTIC THERAPY

Anytime the pulp is exposed or dies, so long as it is not due to extension of periodontal disease or associated with extensive resorption of alveolar bone, there is a need for pulp therapy. The most common indications for veterinary endodontics are (1) broken teeth, (2) pulp exposure due to excessive wear, (3) pulpal hemorrhage, (4) pulp death due to thermal damage or other trauma, (5) reimplantation of avulsed teeth, and (6) tooth transplants (Fig. 2).

In small animal practice, fractured teeth are commonly seen. Unfortunately, many owners and veterinarians ignore fractured teeth in pets. Presumably, this is due to a lack of awareness of the difficulties that the pet will encounter when there has been pulp exposure. Furthermore, the pet will complain very little; thus, its discomfort is often completely overlooked.

Another common cause of pulp disease is excessive wear. This

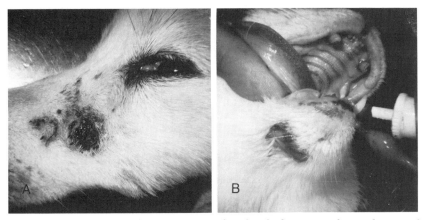

Figure 1. Consequence of not treating a tooth with pulp disease. A, Abscessed carnassial tooth. B, Abscessed canine tooth.

usually occurs when a pet has a chewing vice (rock chewing, gate chewing, and so on) but can also occur with occlusal trauma. When tooth wear is very gradual and the pulp is otherwise healthy, the odontoblasts have the ability to repair and seal the canal by secreting a secondary dentinal substance. This is seen clinically as a tan-colored circle in the middle of a worn-down tooth, much like one would see when aging an older horse by its tooth wear. However, when the pulp becomes diseased and necrotic, this will no longer be a tan color; it will be seen as a dark brown or black.[20]

Teeth that have pulpal hemorrhage due to trauma are another indication for therapy. The affected teeth are usually recognized by their reddish-purple hue. This color change is due to the refraction of the hemoglobin along the dentinal tubules. After a period of weeks or months, these "purple" teeth will turn grey as the pulp necroses and the hemoglobin is broken down. If not treated, these teeth will usually result in apical abscessation, tooth resorption, or avulsion and are therefore good candidates for endodontic therapy.[1, 20]

Other suspected causes of pulp diseases include thermal damage, which can be due to the improper use of ultrasonic scalers, excessive pressure in orthodontic movement, and hematogenous infection. In cases in which there is no external evidence of tooth disease (that is, a normal-looking crown and gingival and periodontal structures), one must rely on clinical signs and radiographs to make the diagnosis. On a radiograph, diseased pulp will not be evident until apical abscessation begins, which is recognized by an area of radiolucency around the apex of the tooth root.[11]

When a tooth has been traumatically avulsed without being fractured, as is the case many times when the pet is hit by a car or

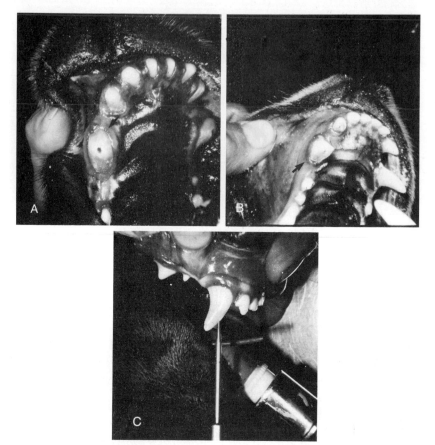

Figure 2. Examples of endodontically diseased teeth that are candidates for root canal therapy. *A,* Exposed pulp due to excessive wear. *B,* Fractured canine tooth. *C,* Pulpal hemorrhage (shaded area on crown in figure), which will be seen as a purplish change in the crown.

kicked by a horse, the missing tooth can be reimplanted with a high degree of success.[1] The avulsion has killed the pulp, however, and the reimplanted tooth must have endodontic treatment either prior to or within a few weeks after reimplantation.

Heterogeneous tooth transplants are possible in fresh or non-periodontically diseased alveolar sockets, although the success rate is considerably less than with a homogeneous tooth reimplantation.[1] Here, too, the donor tooth must be treated endodontically.

CLINICAL SIGNS

It is easy to recognize the pulp disease when a tooth is fractured or has changed color. However, the other clinical signs may be relatively obscure. Occasionally, an owner will report that the pet refuses to chew on bones, toys, or hard foods even though it has done so in the past. Sometimes the pet will be seen chewing on one side only or even acting hungry but refusing to bite down. Some owners have reported seeing a constant licking motion in pets with endodontically diseased teeth. Endodontically diseased teeth are initially sensitive to hot and/or cold, but it is difficult to observe this phenomenon in the normal situation without intentional challenge. When the clinical signs are obscure, one may have to depend upon radiographs to confirm the diagnosis.

PULPOTOMY AND PULP CAPPING VERSUS SURGICAL OR NONSURGICAL ROOT CANAL TECHNIQUES

If the pulp is relatively normal and noninfected, as may be the case with a very fresh tooth fracture (less than 2 hours old), if a crown is cut off to disarm a tooth, or if the pulp cavity is entered while drilling out a carious lesion, it is possible to protect the otherwise healthy pulp and put a filling in the tooth.[6, 20] This is done using pulpotomy and a pulp-capping technique.

When the pulp is grossly contaminated, infected, or dead, as occurs with fractures more than a few hours old, it is best to consider the full endodontic procedure or root canal.[6, 11, 20, 24] The exception to this would be in a very young animal, in which the tooth is just a shell of enamel and a small dentinal layer with a large pulp cavity. If the pulp is not obviously dead or necrotic, it is worth the risk to cap these teeth, in the hope that, even if the pulp eventually dies, there may be additional dentin formation. If the pulp later dies, one must decide to either complete the root canal therapy or extract the tooth.[25]

SURGICAL VERSUS NONSURGICAL ROOT CANAL

A root canal is considered to be surgical when access to the apex of the tooth root is gained by surgical incision and a filling is placed retrograde in the root tip. This is in contrast to the nonsurgical root canal procedure in which the pulp cavity is accessed via the crown only.

The ultimate success of a root canal procedure depends upon obtaining a proper apical seal.[11, 16, 24] When employing a surgical method of endodontic repair, both ends of the tooth are sealed mechanically. However, with the nonsurgical methods, one depends upon the body to complete the apical seal. There are many references in the literature as to which method is preferred.[2, 6, 11, 15–19, 23–25] For practical purposes, including time and relative cost, I prefer to use the nonsurgical or coronal-access-only technique in the majority of my cases. In the following instances, however, I recommend using an apicoectomy and retrograde filling:

1. When there is an obvious apical abscess with dissolution of bone (as determined by radiograph).

2. When I have accidentally broken off a file and it is lodged in the canal.

3. In the rare instance that a simple nonsurgical root canal fails, as evidenced by apical abscessation.

EQUIPMENT

Several kinds of equipment are needed to perform endodontic procedures:

1. Power source and drill to gain access to the canal and prepare the tooth for fillings.

2. Files, broaches, and/or reamers to clean and shape the canal.

3. Flushing solutions for cleansing and disinfecting the canal.

4. Canal drying aids.

5. Filling materials for the canal.

6. Restoration materials for the crown.

7. Instruments for placement of filling materials and restorations.

A variety of power sources are available, but essentially, they must be able to drive a bur at speeds high enough to cut through the enamel. The ultra high-speed (250,000 to 350,000 rpm) air-driven equipment with an automatic water spray works best. However, the slower-speed, higher-torque electric engines will work nicely as long as adequate cooling is used. Round carbide burs probably work best to gain the initial access through the crown, but an inverted cone-type bur that is designed to make an undercut works best to prepare the cavity for a filling, especially where an amalgam restoration is used. Some of the composites will bond to the tooth; therefore, an undercut is not necessary when they are used.

There are basically three types of instruments for cleaning and shaping the pulp canal: barbed broaches, reamers, and files. Barbed broaches are made with spurs that are gouged from the round shaft of the instrument. The shaft is weakened at the base of each spur, making this a fragile instrument that can break off in a canal if twisted or bent excessively.[23] Barbed broaches are very efficient for removal of pulp tissue and necrotic debris from the canal, however.

Reamers and files are made by twisting square or triangular shafts of metal on their long axes. Files receive more turns than do reamers; thus, the cutting edges of files are more horizontal and the filing edges closer together than those of reamers. Because of their design, files are used in a push-pull or in-and-out fashion; reamers work best with a rotary motion, making about a half turn each time it is inserted then withdrawing several millimeters to avoid tension and breakage.[23]

Reamers and files are manufactured in so-called standardized sizes numbered 08 to 140. The size numbers refer to relative graduation in the width of each instrument.[23, 24]

Most reamers and files are manufactured for use in human dentistry and come in lengths of about 25 to 30 mm. These files will work satisfactorily for most teeth in dogs and domestic cats. An exception to this is the dog's canine tooth. Because of the excessive length of the canine tooth, special files or reamers of 40 to 55 mm in length are required. Such instruments are now readily available from manufacturers catering to the veterinary field (Henry Schein Co., for example). While some of these instruments are autoclavable, most files, broaches, and reamers are not; therefore, asepsis is usually maintained by cold sterilization.

For large animals, zoo animals, and exotics, special files or reamers must be custom-made.

The standard flushing solutions include sodium hypochlorite (or Clorox) used half strength, 3 per cent hydrogen peroxide, and sterile water or saline. Sterile paper points and compressed air are used to dry the canal. Dustoff,* which is a canned compressed air source readily available from photo stores and hobby shops, can be used if a compressor is not available.

There are many materials available for filling the canal, and their usage varies widely. The following is a list of some of the most commonly used products.

Materials for Filling Root Canal

1. Silver points
2. Gutta percha points
3. Zinc oxide-eugenol
4. Calcium hydroxide
    A. Root-Cal (Ellman International Manufacturing Inc., Hewlett, New York). A calcium hydroxide paste that is thin, fluid, and free flowing.
    B. Dy-Cal (L. D. Caulk Co., Division of Densply Interna-

---

*Falcon Safety Products, Inc., Mountainside, New Jersey.

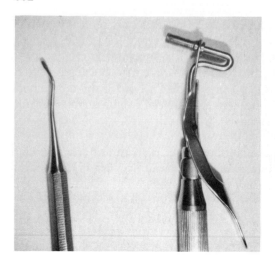

Figure 3. Example of an amalgam carrier and plugger.

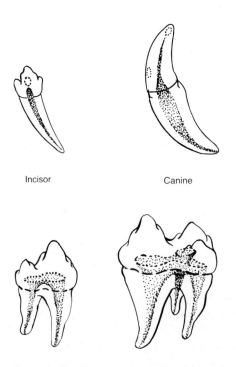

Incisor   Canine

Figure 4. Pulp chambers of single-rooted teeth and the communicating pulp chambers of multirooted teeth.

Double root   Triple root

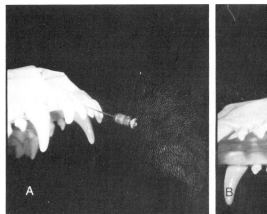
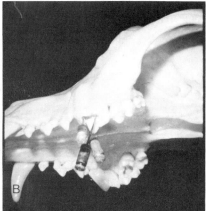
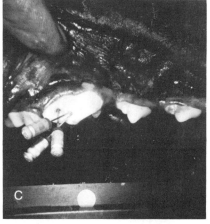

Figure 5. Drill sites for coronal access of a single-rooted tooth versus a multirooted tooth. A, Root canal file in access site for endodontic therapy on incisor (single root). B, Three root canal files showing coronal access necessary for triple-rooted teeth. C, Clinical example of triple-rooted tooth with root canal files in place.

tional Inc., Milford, Delaware). A calcium hydroxide paste that is thick, pasty, and hardens rapidly.
5. I. R. M. (L. D. Caulk Co., Division of Densply International Inc., Milford, Delaware).
6. Life (Kerr Division of Sybron Corp., Romulus, Michigan).

Materials for Filling the Crown

1. Amalgam
   A. Silver and mercury mixed by hand using mortar and pestle.
   B. Pre-mixed capsules. Many brands are available. Two brands are Titan and Cluster, both manufactured by The S. S. White Co., Dental Products International, Phila-

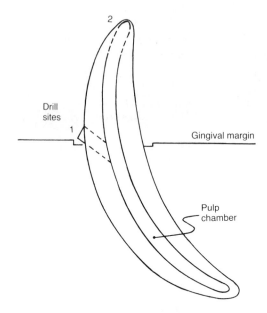

Figure 6. Diagram of canine tooth showing the two drill sites needed to perform root canal therapy on this long, curved tooth.

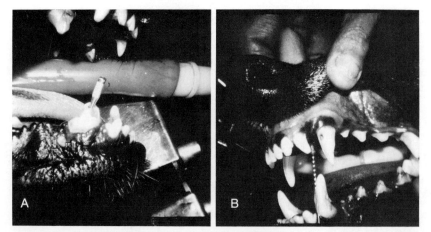

Figure 7. A, Root canal file inserted into pulp chamber of fractured canine tooth. B, File being withdrawn with pulp tissue.

delphia, Pennsylvania. When using the pre-mixed capsules, it is necessary to have an amalgamator to shake
and properly mix the ingredients within the capsule.

One needs an amalgam carrier, which is a smaller
instrument designed to gather amalgam into the barrel
and then deliver it into the preparation by depressing
the lever above the barrel. Condensers (pluggers) are
needed to pack the material firmly into the site, making
sure that the undercut is completely filled. Carvers or
shaping instruments can then be used to smooth and
contour the surface. (Fig. 3).

2. Composites
   A. Chemically activated
      1. Concise (3M, St. Paul, Minnesota)
      2. Adaptic (Johnson & Johnson Products Inc. New Bruns-
         wick, New Jersey)
      3. Compolite (Super Dent, Mfg. for Rugby Laboratories
         Inc., Rockville Center, New York)
   B. Photo-cured
      1. Nuva-lite (L. D. Caulk Co., Division of Densply
         International Inc., Milford, Delaware)
      2. Mistique (Johnson & Johnson Products Inc., New
         Brunswick, New Jersey)
   In order to use the photo-cured composites, it is necessary
   to have the special ultraviolet light source required to
   activate these restoratives.

BASIC STEPS FOR PERFORMING PULP THERAPY

Once pulp therapy is chosen for a diseased tooth, the first step
is to place the patient under general anesthesia. All of the teeth
should then be cleaned and polished to rid the teeth of plaque and
calculus. In order to achieve asepsis, the teeth and mouth are then
disinfected. The next step is to gain access to the pulp cavity. In the
case of a fractured tooth, the access may already be present. When
disarming canine teeth, the crown is amputated using a diamond
disc; otherwise, the enamel and dentin must be drilled to gain the
necessary access to the pulp. Most teeth can be treated endodontically through a single site drilled into the crown. However, it should
be noted that:

1. Multirooted teeth have a pulp chamber that communicates
between all roots; therefore, if one root is treated, all roots and the
coronal part of the pulp must also be treated (Figs. 4 and 5).

2. With the large, curved canine tooth, a double entry is usually

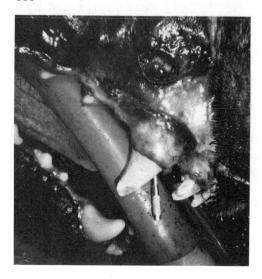

Figure 8. Surgical root canal of maxillary canine tooth showing approach for amputation of apex of tooth root.

necessary in order to perform the root canal procedure. One site is at the tip of the crown and a second at the gingival margin (Fig. 6)

Once adequate access is gained in the case in which pulp capping is indicated, the coronal part of the pulp is carefully removed and a buffer material is placed over the remaining vital pulp, the access is prepared to receive a filling, and then the filling is put in place.

With a nonsurgical root canal, the pulp cavity must be thoroughly filed and cleansed of all organic debris. This is done by using root canal files, broaches, and/or reamers of subsequently larger gauges (diameter) until nothing but clean dentinal shavings are removed and the canal has been shaped in a funnel-like fashion that is wider at the coronal access (Fig. 7). This allows for ease of installing and condensing the root canal filling materials.[22] Throughout the procedure, the canal is flushed clean and disinfected. Finally, it is rinsed and dried. At that time, the canal can be filled and a restoration (filling) placed in the crown.

In the case requiring a surgical root canal, the procedure is exactly the same except that once the canal has been filed clean, it is measured and an incision is made in the mucosa above the apex of the root. The bone is drilled away and the apex of the tooth is amputated (Fig. 8). Thus, a retrograde filling can be put in place prior to the filling of the canal. The mucosal flap is then sutured back in place, and the completion of the procedure is just the same as for the nonsurgical method.

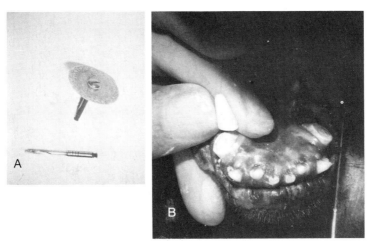

Figure 9. A, A diamond disk. B, Amputated crown of disarmed canine tooth.

TECHNIQUE FOR PULP CAPPING

First access to the pulp chamber must be gained through the crown. When disarming teeth, this is done by amputation of the crown using a safe-side diamond disk (Fig. 9). For a case involving a fresh fracture, the exposure is already made. Then the coronal part of the pulp is carefully and antiseptically removed. This is accomplished by using a pulp evacuator or drill. Hemorrhage must then be controlled. This can be done using the very light pressure of an epinephrine-soaked cotton pellet placed over the remaining vital pulp.[6] Next, enlarge the coronal end of the pulp chamber with a round bur to a depth of about 4 mm. Then use an inverted cone bur to undercut and carve a seat for a thermal insulation layer. A calcium hydroxide product (For example, Dy-Cal*) works best for this buffer layer.[4, 6] A simple and inexpensive way to assist in the application of buffer materials is the use of Jiffy Cement Tubes.† They are hollow, plastic tubes that are open at both ends but taper to a fine point at one end. The calcium hydroxide (or any paste-consistency material) can be scooped up into the tube through the large open end. Then, by plugging that end with a cotton pellet or fingertip, the tube can be squeezed, thereby delivering the material through the narrowed end in a fine application. After allowing a minute or two for drying, drill away any excess buffer material, then follow with a layer of zinc phosphate cement or an intermediate restorative material (I.R.M.,* for example). This establishes a firm backing for the final filling.

---

*L. D. Caulk Co., Division of Dansply International Inc., Milford, Delaware.
†Teledyne Getz, Elk Grove Village, Illinois.

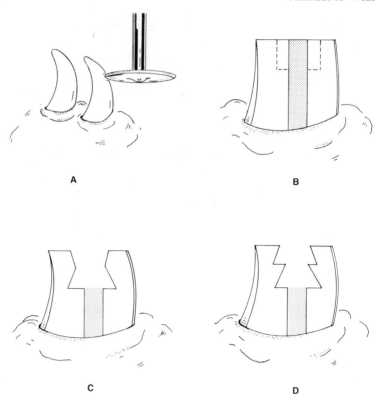

Figure 10. Steps in disarming and pulp capping canine teeth. *A*, Diamond disk being used to amputate crown of canine tooth. *B*, Drill site to remove coronal part of vital pulp. *C*, Undercut to retain thermal buffer (calcium hydroxide). *D*, Undercut to retain filling.

Using the inverted cone bur, the coronal end of the canal is now undercut to prepare for the filling. Care should be taken to ensure that the undercut does not thin the lateral wall excessively; however, a good taper of 1 to 2 mm is necessary to hold an amalgam filling in place (Fig. 10). When a composite resin filling is to be used, the taper may be less important, because some of these products will chemically bond to the dentin. When using composites, the tooth is now ready for the filling; however, if an amalgam filling is to be used, the undercut area should be coated with a dentin tubular sealer such as Compolite.* Once dry, the tooth is then ready for the amalgam filling. It is important to use an amalgam carrier to pick up and place this filling material into the defect. It should then be packed thoroughly in place with amalgam pluggers and molded to the contour of the tooth. One must allow the amalgam to dry before polishing. Because the hardening takes a minimum of 1 hour,

---

*Super Dent, Mfg. for Ruggy Laboratories Inc., Rockville Center, New York.

it is preferable that polishing be done after 24 hours. That usually means another office visit and an anesthetic procedure, if the animal is excitable or unruly. Often, therefore, the polishing of an amalgam filling is not done until the next prophylaxis treatment. A pet should be fed soft food only for at least 24 hours after receiving an amalgam filling.

TECHNIQUE FOR NONSURGICAL ROOT CANAL

The basic steps for performing a root canal procedure were outlined previously. Although many variations in technique are described in the literature,[2, 6, 11, 15–19, 23–25] the following description is my procedure of choice. It has been used with greater than 90 per cent clinical success involving hundreds of cases over the past 10 years.

As with all endodontic procedures, the first step is gaining access to the pulp via the crown. This part of the technique has been described previously. Next, the root canal is probed using a very small gauge file (no. 15 or 20) in order to seek out the direction and limits of the pulp cavity. It is best to radiograph at this point to ensure that the file has gone into the canal and extended to the depth without penetrating or breaking through the apex. The file is then marked with a rubber stopper, or a measurement is taken to reference the proper depth. (*Note*: If the file does not come with a rubber marker, one can cut a small piece of rubber band, pierce it with the file, then move it along the shaft to mark the canal depth.)

Once the proper depth has been determined, the canal is cleaned and enlarged. This is accomplished by inserting the small gauge file or reamer to just within a millimeter of the tip, then twisting and withdrawing to extract the pulp material. Note that the success of the procedure is placed in greater jeopardy when materials penetrate the apex than when they have not gone quite far enough—that is, it is better to file a little short than to file too long.[22] The file should not be rotated more than about 90 degrees or else it may break off in the canal. This procedure is repeated with files with successively larger gauges until all the pulp is removed. One can tell when all the pulp has been removed when nothing but clean dentinal shavings are withdrawn.

While the pulp is being removed, the canal is shaved into a funnel shape as the files are withdrawn against the wall in a circular fashion.

Throughout the procedure, the files can be lubricated, as the removal of debris and disinfection are aided by the periodic flushing of the canal. This is accomplished by using syringes with 20- or 23-

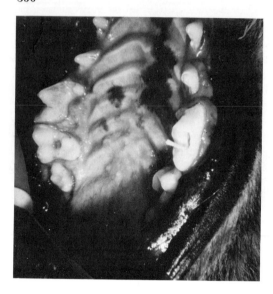

Figure 11. Paper point being used to dry pulp chamber.

gauge needles containing 50 per cent solution of sodium hypochlorite (household bleach), hydrogen peroxide, and normal saline and flushing in that same order.

Once cleansed of all organic pulp tissue and debris, the canal must be dried in preparation for the filling materials. This is done by using sterile paper points that are inserted into the canal to the apex, then withdrawn (Fig. 11). This is repeated until all moisture is absorbed (when the paper point that is withdrawn is perfectly dry). This drying process can be hastened by the careful use of compressed air. A gentle puff of air directed down the canal will blow away the moisture and speed evaporation. Care should be taken to not force the air through the apical foramen.

Now we are ready to fill the canal. I prefer to use calcium hydroxide products, because they have been shown to effect an apical seal while retarding any tendency for root resorption,[5, 9, 12, 27] together with gutta percha points, which are inert, rubber-like cones. They are used to eliminate air pockets and filling defects when condensed or compacted into the canal. Because of the ease of administration, I use either Hypo-cal* or Root-Cal.* They come packaged in a syringe-like container with a long, blunt, needle-like tip. By inserting the tip into the canal, then screwing in the plunger, it will deliver the fluid calcium hydroxide to the apex. Continue to inject the material as the tip is withdrawn. This leaves the canal mostly filled with the calcium hydroxide. Then select a gutta percha

*Ellman International Manufacturing Inc., Hewlett, New York.

point that approximates the size of the largest gauge file that was used to ream the canal. Using aseptic technique, gently push the gutta percha point to the depth of the canal. The gutta percha point is cut so that its length is such that, when inserted to the apex, it comes 2 to 3 mm short of reaching the coronal access, thus allowing room for the undercutting and placement of the filling. With this first gutta percha point in place, condense it laterally by inserting a long pointed spreader using firm pressure. After withdrawing the spreader, insert another, usually smaller gauge, gutta percha point, cut off the excess, and continue the process until the spreader will no longer move, indicating that the canal is completely filled and condensed. At this point, we are ready to place an intermediate restorative and filling as previously described.

TECHNIQUE FOR SURGICAL ROOT CANAL

For those cases in which a surgical root canal is indicated, proceed exactly as previously mentioned up to the point that the canal has been filed clean. Using a file inserted to the depth of the root to serve as a measurement, place the file adjacent to the tooth in order to mark the point of the incision. Incise the mucous membrane over the estimated position of the tooth apex. In mandibular canines, however, it is easier to make an incision through the skin over the ventral aspect of the mandible and beneath the first premolar at a point determined by using the length of the tooth as marked on the root canal file. Using a periosteal elevator, reflect all soft tissue down to subperiosteal bone. Again using the mark on the root canal file to determine the point of the apex of the tooth, drill away the bone with a round bur and expose at least 3 to 4 mm of the tip of the tooth. With the same bur, amputate the apex. Then, with an inverted cone bur, undercut to prepare for an amalgam filling that is placed in the site using a retrograde carrier and pluggers. With the root filling in place, the soft tissues are sutured back over the defect using a 2-0 or 3-0 chromic gut. From this point, the rest of the root canal procedure is exactly the same as the nonsurgical method, including the filling of the crown as previously described.

RESULTS

The results will certainly vary according to which technique is used, what materials are employed, and the experience of the practitioner. However, once the technique is mastered, it will take a mere 10 to 15 minutes to perform a root canal procedure on a simple incisor and probably no more than 1 hour to 1½ hours for a difficult canine or carnassial tooth. The long-term success rate has been demonstrated as being quite high. In most cases, one would expect an endodontically treated tooth to last the lifetime of the pet.[1, 3, 7, 10, 11, 24]

SUMMARY

It is known that pets with broken teeth or teeth with other diseases of the pulp suffer considerable pain and frequent infection. To ignore these problem teeth would not only be inhumane, it would risk chronic infection, abscessation, and tooth loss.

Although extraction of these teeth is sometimes necessary, the procedure is often difficult to perform and painful for the animal. The resultant tooth loss is cosmetically displeasing and, frequently, there is compromise in function.

The endodontic treatment of these teeth, on the other hand, is relatively easy to perform. It almost always results in immediate cessation of pain and will usually allow the tooth to remain functional for the lifetime of the pet.

REFERENCES

1. Beard, G.: Personal communication, 1979.
2. Bellizze, R., et al.: Non-surgical endodontic therapy, utilizing lingual coronal access on the mandibular canine tooth of dogs. J. Am. Vet. Med. Assoc., 179:370–374, 1981.
3. Colmery, B.: American Veterinary Dental Society Meeting, Las Vegas, Nevada, 1981.
4. Dannerberg, J. L.: Pedodontic endodontics. Dent. Clin. North Am., 18(2):367–377, 1977.
5. Dylenshi, J. J.: Apical closure of immature pulpless teeth in monkeys. Oral Surg., 33:438–449, 1972.
6. Eisenmenger, E., and Zetner, K.: Veterinary Dentistry. Philadelphia, Lea & Febiger, 1985, pp. 84–98.
7. Emily, P.: Non-Surgical Endodontics. Notes from Vetodontics Lecture #3. Fort Collins, Colorado State University.
8. Glick, D. H.: Interrelationship of systemic and endodontic clinical problems. Dent. Clin. North Am., 18:(2):233, 1974.
9. Goldman, M.: Root-end closure techniques including apexification. Dent. Clin. North Am., 18(2):297–303, 1974.
10. Harvey, C.: Oral disease and veterinary dentistry. In Proceedings of the Seminar Presented to Greater Cincinnati Veterinary Medical Association, May 1985.
11. Harvey, C. E.: Veterinary Dentistry. Philadelphia, W. B. Saunders Co., 1985, pp. 86–96.
12. Ham, J. W., et al.: Induced apical closure of immature pulpless teeth in monkeys. Oral Surg., 33:438–449, 1972.
13. Langeland, K.: Root canal sealants and pastes. Dent. Clin. North Am. 18(2):309–327, 1974.
14. Luebhe, R. G.: Surgical endodontics. Dent. Clin. North Am., 18(2):379–382, 1977.

15. Ridgeway, R. L., and Zelke, D. R.: Non-surgical endodontic techniques for dogs. J. Am. Vet. Med. Assoc., *174*(1):83–85, 1976.
16. Ross, D. L.: A partial reconstruction technique for canine teeth. Pract. Vet., *43*(1):46–48, 1971.
17. Ross, D. L.: Canine endodontic therapy. J. Am. Vet. Med. Assoc., *180*:356–357, 1981.
18. Ross, D. L., and Myers, J. W.: Endodontic therapy for canine teeth in the dog. J. Am. Vet. Med. Assoc., *157*:1713–1718, 1970.
19. Rubin, L. D., Maplesden, D.C., and Singer, R. R.: Root canal therapy in dogs. Vet. Med. Small Anim. Clin., *73*(5):593–598, 1978.
20. Saidla, J.: Notes on Endodontics. Auburn, Alabama, April 1979, pp. 28–32.
21. Sargenti. Endodontics: Efficient Endodontics for Every Day Practice. A.E.S. Seminars—Eastern. Levittown, Pennsylvania.
22. Schilder, H.: Shaping and cleaning the root canal. Dent. Clin. North Am. *18*(2):1974.
23. Schmeltzer, L. D., Carolan, R. J., and Ohfa, R. M.: Use of conventional endodontic therapy in a case of veterinary medicine. J. Am. Dent. Assoc., *100*:218–219, 1980.
24. Tholen, M. A.: Concepts in Veterinary Dentistry. Edwardsville, Kansas, Veterinary Medicine Publishing Co., 1983, pp. 114–132.
25. Tholen, M.: Veterinary endodontics. J. Am. Vet. Med. Assoc., *180*:4–6, 1981.
26. Torneck, C. D.: Biologic effects of endodontic procedures on developing incisor teeth: Effect of partial and total pulp removal. Oral Surg., *30*:258–261, 1970.
27. Van Hassel, H. J.: Induction of foraminal closure. J. Can. Dent. Assoc., *35*:606–608, 1969.

Blue Cross Animal Hospital
8429 Lee Highway
Fairfax, Virginia 22031

Dentistry   0195–5616/86 $0.00 + .20

Restorative Dentistry

*Peter Emily, D.D.S.**

Owing to the extensive amount of material, methods, and techniques used in restorative dentistry and the amount of research that has been done, it is impossible to cover this subject in such a short article. We wish to cover as much of the subject as possible in order to stimulate the reader to further his or her own reading and research into this field and to develop his or her own skills and techniques.

Restorative dentistry is the restoration of a tooth and its function as close as possible to its normal and natural state prior to disease or trauma. It is not limited to the restoration of dental caries (decay) only. Because the incidence of dental caries (decay) is less than 7 per cent in dogs and only slightly higher in cats, the restoration of fractured teeth after root canal therapy, enamel bonding for enamel defects or erosion, and the replacement of trauma-induced enamel fractures are the primary focus of restorative dentistry. The enamel organ is the only protection the tooth has from decay.

The demineralization of enamel is an inorganic breakdown of the enamel cuticle. The carious breakdown of dentin is of an organic nature and is much more rapid than the enamel demineralization. Exposed root structure has no enamel covering and is very susceptible to decay and external resorption as seen in gum line defects in cats.

No restorative material presently available is as good as supported tooth structure, and it is unlikely that a usable dental restorative material with the physical properties of enamel will ever be developed. The purpose of cavity preparation is to remove carious material and preserve sound tooth structure. Any additional removal of tooth structure is necessary for the convenience of the operator or because of limitations of the restorative materials. There is no specific ideal design for cavity preparation. Each defect should be custom-designed to remove the caries or defect and perform the

---

*Director and Chief of Animal Dentistry, Colorado State University, College of Veterinary Medicine and Biomedical Sciences, Fort Collins, Colorado

additional steps necessitated by the limitations of the operator or restorative material.[15]

NOMENCLATURE AND ARMAMENTARIUM

NAMES OF TOOTH SURFACES

The surfaces of a tooth take their name from the oral structure to which they are related.

Occlusal. Pertaining to the masticating surfaces of the posterior teeth.

Buccal. Pertaining to or adjacent to the cheek.

Lingual. Next to or toward the tongue.

Incisal. Relating to the cutting edge of the anterior teeth, the incisors, or cuspids.

Labial. Of or pertaining to a lip or toward the lip.

Mesial. Toward the center line of the dental arch (incisors).

Distal. Away from the median sagittal plane of the face following the curvature of the dental arch (incisors).

Facial. A general term to include buccal and labial surfaces of teeth in both the maxillary and mandibular arches.

Rostral. On the long axis of the tooth, toward the nose (canines, premolars, molars).

Caudal. Toward the tail (canines, premolars, molars).

Proximal. The surface of a tooth or the portion of a cavity that is nearest to the adjacent tooth. The rostral or caudal surface of a tooth.[1]

COMPONENTS OF A CAVITY PREPARATION

Cavity wall. One of the enclosing sides of a prepared cavity. It takes the name of the surface of the tooth adjoining the surface involved and toward which it is placed (for example, the buccal wall of the occlusal cavity preparation is the enclosing side that is toward the buccal surface of the tooth, and the lingual wall of the proximal portion of a cavity preparation is the enclosing side that is toward the lingual surface of the tooth.

Enamel wall. The portion of the wall of a prepared cavity that consists of enamel.

Dentin wall. The portion of the wall of a prepared cavity that consists of dentin.

Axial wall. A wall lying in the direction of the long axis of the tooth.

Pulpal wall. A wall lying in relation to the pulp.

Undercut. The portion of a prepared cavity confined by walls that coverge toward the surface. A localized channel within a cavity preparation (not linear).

Margin. The junction of the wall of the cavity with the surface of the tooth.

Approximal (approximating). Contiguous, adjacent, next to each other.

Cavity debridement. Removal of all debris from a completed cavity preparation by mechanical methods.

Gingival. Pertaining to or in relation to the gingiva.

Interproximal. Between the proximal surfaces of adjoining teeth.

Long axis. An imaginary line passing longitudinally through the center of the body. (In an incisoapical or occlusoapical direction when related to teeth.)

Pulpal. Relating to the pulp or the pulp cavity.

Restoration of cusps. (Preferred to tipping, capping, or shoeing cusps.) The reduction and inclusion of cusps within a cavity preparation and their restoration to functional occlusion with restorative material.[1]

GENERAL CONSIDERATIONS

The following are rules of cavity preparation and restoration that must be considered:

1. Removal of caries without weakening tooth structure.

2. Extension of a cavity preparation to remove all undermined and carious enamel and dentin.

3. Design of cavity preparation to facilitate filling, and finishing of preparation to minimize the weak points of the filling material.

4. The preservation of a maximum amount of tooth structure retaining the inherent strength contained in a tooth.[7]

The preceding rules hold true not only for the removal of caries but also for the restoration of a broken cusp or filling of access sites of an endodontically treated tooth.

A human classification of dental caries will define the types and sites of decay or areas to be restored after trauma or erosion.

Classification of cavities is the intention to group together in classes, cavities (decay) that require a similar line of treatment in order that these may be more closely associated.

Class I. Cavities beginning in structural defects in the teeth pits and fissures. These are located in the occlusal surfaces of the premolars and molars, in the occlusal two thirds of the buccal surfaces of the molars, in the lingual surfaces of the upper incisors, and occasionally in the lingual surfaces of the upper molars (Fig. 1A).

Class II. Cavities in the proximal surfaces of the premolars and molars (rarely seen in dogs and cats) (Fig. 1B).

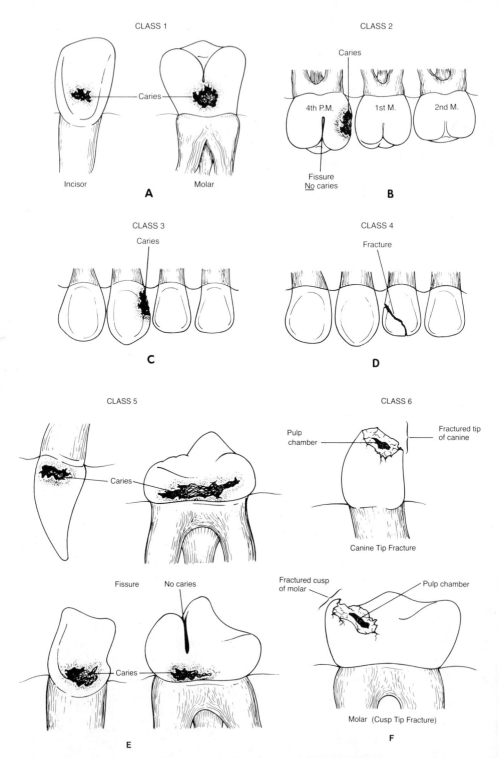

Figure 1. *A* to *F*, Classification of cavities/defects.

Class III. Cavities in the proximal surfaces of the incisors and canines that do not involve the removal and restoration of the incisal angle (rarely seen in cats and dogs) (Fig. 1C).

Class IV. Cavities in the proximal surfaces of the incisers and canines that do require the removal and restoration of the incisal angle (common in fractures of front teeth) (Fig. 1D).

Class V. Cavities in the gingival third—not pit cavities—of the labial buccal or lingual surfaces of the teeth (second most common type of cavity in dogs and cats) (Fig. 1E).

Class VI. Defect on the incisal edges of anterior teeth or the cusp tips of posterior teeth (this is the most common type of cavity the veterinarian will deal with). An example would be fractured cusp tips on canines and molars (Fig. 1F).

Classes II, III, and IV are all smooth surface cavities. They all occur in positions in which the surfaces of the teeth are habitually unclean.[1]

ANATOMY

A review of basic dental anatomy is necessary to familiarize the practitioner with the relationships of enamel to dentin and the pulpal tissues (Fig. 2).

Enamel is the inorganic component covering the coronal aspect of the tooth. Enamel rods run at right angles to the tooth surface and are important in that any unsupported enamel at the surface of a restoration (that is, edges or portions of unsupported or undermined enamel rods) will break off in a short time, leaving a defect or void at the junction of the tooth and restoration. This will trap food and debris, leading to a breakdown of the restoration. A simple scraping of the cavity preparation walls with the edges of a sharp spoon excavator will remove these unsupported enamel rods prior to placement of the restoration. The depth of dentin must be visualized while cavity preparation is being performed. The dentin protects the pulp from thermal shock and restorative material irritation. Whenever cavity preparation or caries is so extensive that it encroaches upon the pulp, an insulating base must be placed over the pulpal wall to protect the pulp chamber from irritation and eventual pulpal necrosis. (See Pulp Treatments.)

A large percentage of defects seen in veterinary dentistry, especially in cats, occurs below the cementoenamel junction (the junction of crown and root). Without the protection of enamel, the root surface is very susceptible to decay or external resorption. The cavity preparation is made directly into root structure or dentin; therefore, precaution of undermined or unsupported enamel is not needed, for this procedure is entirely in dentin (Fig. 3).

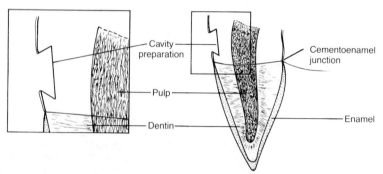

Figure 2. A schematic drawing of the basic anatomy of a tooth and its supporting structure. Note the distance of the pulp chamber and canal from the surface and the depth and thickness of the dentin. Note also that the enamel rods are at right angles to the dentin and the tooth surface. These relationships must be remembered whenever restorative dentistry is needed to prevent pulpal exposure and to perfect the best retention and finish of the restoration.

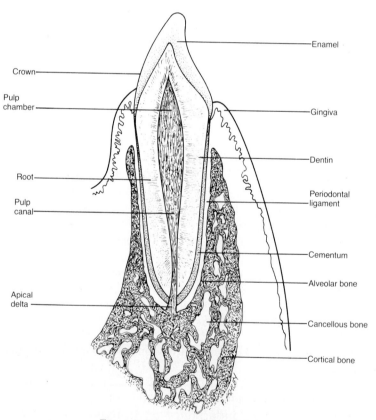

Figure 3. Preparation of root defect.

EQUIPMENT

Several types of dental units are available to the veterinary profession. These range in price and function from a simple dremmel tool to a sophisticated air-driven dental handpiece.

A list of these units follows:

1. *Dremmel tool.* Very inexpensive, but it can be used. It is difficult to control with accuracy and is capable of 5000 to 6000 rpm.

2. *Electric belt-driven triple arm and handpiece bench unit.* A reasonable and functional unit. It is not very fast, but it possesses much torque and is excellent for dental prophylaxis (Fig. 4). It is capable of 10,000 to 20,000 rpm.

3. *Electric dental engine and handpiece.* Very good for both dental restoration and prophylaxis. It is capable of 15,000 to 30,000 rpm. (See picture in Schein catalog, number 100-2787, VC-50 Dental Care unit.*)

4. *Air-turbine handpiece.* Both slow- and high-speed handpieces are air-driven. They are the most expensive units. They deliver very high speeds to the high-speed handpiece and are extremely efficient in removing tooth structure. The slow-speed handpiece, such as the Midwest Shorty,† is as efficient as the electric or belt-driven unit for prophylaxis or any procedure when slow speed in needed. It is capable of 150,000 to 300,000 rpm in high speed (Fig. 5A and B).

Burs

There are extensive combinations and types of dental burs available to do any and all forms of restorative dentistry. In time, the practitioner will find those that fit his or her desires best.

Bur. A rotary cutting instrument of steel or tungsten carbide that is supplied with cutting heads of various shapes and two or more sharp-edged blades. It is used as a rotary grinder.

Cross-cut bur. A bur with blades slotted perpendicular to the axis of the bur.

Finishing bur. A bur with numerous, fine-cutting blades placed close together. It is used to contour metallic restorations.

Inverted cone bur. A bur with a head shaped like a truncated cone, the larger diameter being at the terminal or distal end.

Round bur. A bur with a sphere-shaped head.

Plain-cut fissure bur. A bur without cross-cuts that has a cylinder-shaped head.

---

*Henry Schein, Inc., Port Washington, New York.
†Midwest, Des Plaines, Illinois

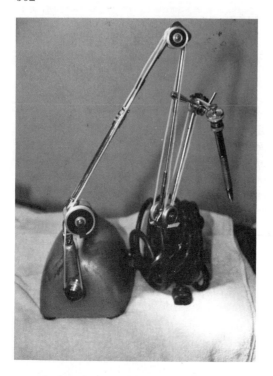

Figure 4. Electric belt-driven, triple-arm dental unit.

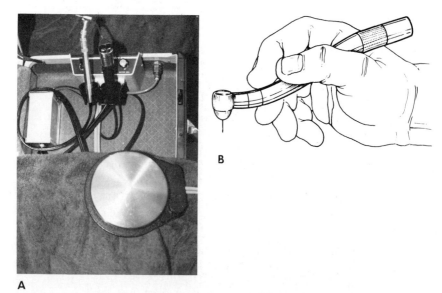

B

A

Figure 5. *A*, Air-turbine dental unit with high-speed handpiece and three-way syringe. *B*, Pen grasp for maximum control of dental handpiece.

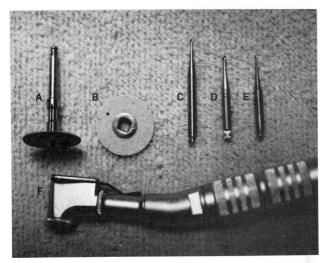

Figure 6. Latch-type burs. *A*, Sandpaper disk and mandrel latch-type bur. *B*, Sandpaper disk. *C*, No. 1 round latch-type bur. *D*, No. 2 round latch-type, short-shank carbide bur. *E*, No. 1 round latch-type, short-shank bur. *F*, Latch-type contra-angle attachments for use with slow-speed dental units.

Tapered fissure bur. A bur with a long head with sides that converge from the shank to a blunt end.[1]

Burs are available in latch-type for the slow-speed handpiece and contra-angle attachment (Fig. 6) and friction grip for the air-turbine handpiece (Fig. 7). Burs are available in carbon steel and

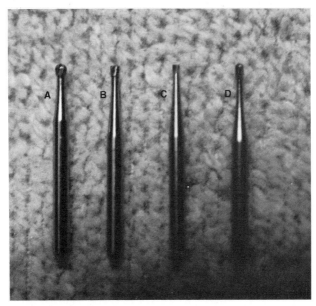

Figure 7. Friction-grip cutting burs. *A*, No. 2 round bur. *B*, No. 35 inverted-cone bur. *C*, No. 34 inverted-cone bur. *D*, No. 330 bur.

tungsten carbide for the air-turbine, contra-angle, and straight hand-pieces.[2]

The most useful dental burs for cutting and enamel reduction are the inverted-cone type (see Fig. 7) (sizes 34 and 35), a round bur (sizes 1 and 2), and pear-shaped 330 burs. For gross reduction of enamel, a straight-fissure bur (sizes 556 and 557) works well. [The finishing of composite restorations and the smoothing of broken and rough edges of enamel are accomplished with finishing and diamond burs, 8-bladed to 20-bladed finishing bur (size 7802), Midwest 12-blade (cone shape) size 7205 and (egg-shaped) 7406,* or bullet-shaped diamond (bur size, Healthco 700-10F or Premier† 700 11 VF) (Fig. 8).]

COMMON EQUIPMENT FOR RESTORATIVE WORK

The following equipment is necessary for performing dental restorations:

1. *Explorer.* A slender, circular, cross-sectioned instrument, tapered to an extremely sharp point for exploring hard-tissue defects. It is available in many shapes.

2. *Mouth mirror.* To aid in seeing the palatal and lingual surfaces.

---

*Healthco
†Premier Dental Products Co., Norristown, Pennsylvania.

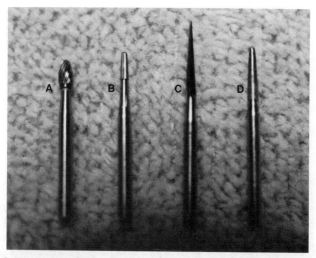

Figure 8. Friction-grip finishing burs for use in high-speed handpiece. *A,* Twelve-bladed bullet-shaped. *B,* Eight-bladed tapered round nose. *C,* Eight-bladed extra long pointed. *D,* Tapered fine-cut diamond.

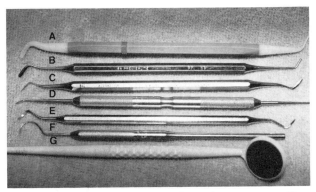

Figure 9. Instrument set-up for restorative work. *A*, Plastic composite filling instrument. *B*, Premierlite PFI W3 filling instrument. *C*, S. S. White Hollenback carver 1–2. *D*, Starlight M-G 89-92 carver. *E*, American Dental 11 7 14 4 0.41 spoon excavator. *F*, Starlite M-G 23 explorer. *G*, Mouth mirror.

3. *Spoon excavator.* A paired hand instrument intended primarily to remove carious material from a cavity; lateral cutting blade is curette-shaped, discoid-shaped, or spoon-shaped, and the entire periphery is sharpened.

4. *Plastic instrument.* An instrument used to manipulate a composite restorative material (Fig. 9).

5. *Silver amalgam carvers.* An instrument used to shape filling material (Fig. 10).

6. *Silver amalgam carriers.* An instrument used to transport amalgam to cavity preparation.

7. *Silver amalgam pluggers.* (Also called condensers.) An instrument or device used to compact or condense a restorative material into a prepared cavity (Fig. 11).

8. *Calcium hydroxide.* A lining for the pulpal wall. (See Pulp Treatments.)

9. *Cavity linear or varnish.* (See Pulp Treatments.)

10. *Size 34 or 35 inverted-cone bur.*

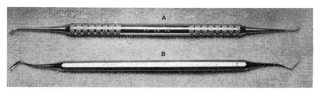

Figure 10. Silver amalgam carvers. *A*, Healthco 89-92 CD carver. *B*, S. S. White Hollenback carver 1–2.

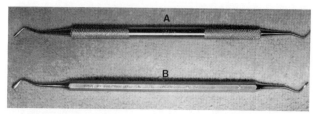

Figure 11. Silver amalgam pluggers. *A*, Rugby Eames no. 1 alloy plugger. *B*, S. S. White HAC no. 3 alloy plugger.

11. *Silver amalgam.* Pellet form preferred.

12. *Composite.* Small particle size, chemical-cured, or light-cured. (See Composite Filling Material.)

13. *Finishing burs.* For composite restoration only.

14. *Sandpaper disks.* Abrasive disk with sandpaper as the abrading medium.

15. *Mandrel.* A shaft that supports or holds an object to be rotated. An instrument, held in a handpiece, that holds a disk, stone, or cup used for grinding, smoothing, or polishing[1] (Fig. 12).

The following is a general step-by-step procedure that can be used for the majority of restorations of a carious or traumatic nature—that is, the closing of an entry for endodontics, the repair of fractured cusps, or the restoration of a carious or resorptive lesion.

Isolate the tooth to be prepared with cotton rolls or gauze sponges to keep it free of saliva and debris.

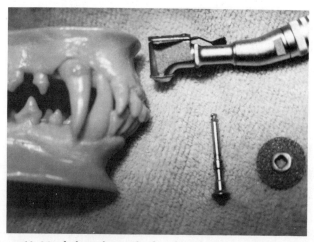

Figure 12. Mandrel attachment for dental handpiece with sandpaper disk.

After proper isolation of the tooth to be prepared, the initial opening of the carious lesion is made with the size 34 or 35 inverted-cone bur to the dentin at the dentinoenamel junction (Figs. 13, 14, and 15).

The preparation is extended to the proximal, incisal, and gingival limits of the carious lesion to establish the form of the cavity outline.

The remainder of the caries is removed with the inverted-cone bur or, if the lesion is extensive, with a hand instrument (the spoon excavator, for example). The dentin may be stained by the caries itself, making it difficult to determine if the caries has been removed. If the dentin has a hard, shiny appearance, even though it is stained and dark from the carious lesion, it is probable that the caries removal is total.

All unsupported enamel or dentin should be removed with a spoon excavator by lightly planing the cavity walls. Retention and undercuts are placed into the dentin with a no. 1 round bur or inverted-cone bur for filling material retention. If caries has extended to or near the pulp, a medicated base of calcium hydroxide is placed over the exposed pulp before a filling material is placed into the cavity. Also, all cavity preparations should be lined or based with cavity varnish for silver amalgam restorations or calcium hydroxide for composite restorations before the final filling material is placed to prevent pulpal pathology, sensitivity from filling material irritation, or toxicity (see Pulp Treatments).

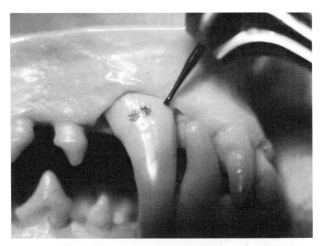

Figure 13. Shaded area on lateral surface of model canine tooth represents a carious lesion.

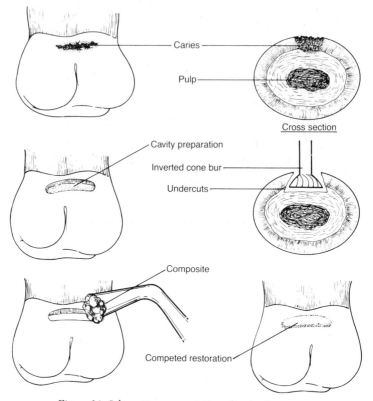

Figure 14. Schematic representation of a simple restoration.

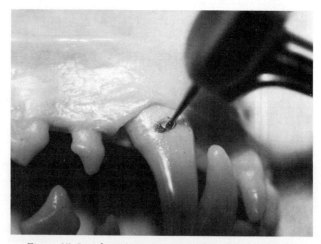

Figure 15. Initial cavity preparation with inverted-cone bur.

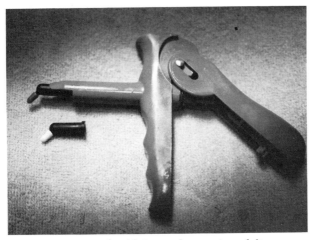

Figure 16. Precapsulated light-cured composite and dispenser.

COMPOSITE FILLING MATERIAL

Composite filling material is manufactured by a number of dental manufacturing companies. Of the various types of composite, two types differentiated by density or particle size are the most practical for restorative use. These are available in chemical-cured and light-cured forms. The light-cured form is the composite of choice because it provides for infinite working time before the light source or curing light is used to polymerize or cure the composite. Light-cured composite is dispensed in many ways, such as Caulk's Prisma,* a precapsulated light-cured composite (Fig. 16). It is ideal for the lamination or bonding procedures in cases of enamel hypoplasia or erosion. A light source, such as Denmat's Visar 2,† is an excellent light-source system. These laminates are used in conjunction with an enamel acid etch technique prior to placement of the composite. This technique will be discussed in detail in the section on cavity preparation and filling.

Chemical-cured composite is made by a number of manufacturer's, such as Healthco, and the manufacturer's instructions should be closely followed. This technique involves the mixing of two parts—a base and a catalyst paste. The two pastes are placed on a paper mixing pad in equal amounts. At the time of mixing, an opaquer may be added to lighten the color or shade of the composite. Canine teeth are whiter than the shades provided by the manufac-

*L. D. Caulk Co., Division of Densply International Inc., Milford, Delaware.
†Denmat, Santa Maria, California.

turer of their human products. The amount of the paste mix should be slightly larger than the approximate amount needed to fill the cavity preparation. The mix is placed into the cavity preparation with a plastic filling instrument (Fig. 17). The plastic instrument prevents the tarnishing of some types of composite material caused by a metal instrument. The composite is condensed or spatulated into the clean, thoroughly dried cavity preparation and undercuts, slightly overfilled, and allowed to set (approximately 2 to 4 minutes) (Fig. 18). After it is set or cured, the composite is finished with the use of the 8- to 20-bladed finishing burs or diamond finishing burs (Fig. 19) and a sandpaper disk and mandrel in the slow-speed handpiece using the latch-type dental contra-angle attachment (Fig. 20A and B).

AMALGAM

Amalgam is an alloy of silver and mercury with small amounts of other metals. Copper amalgam alloy is also available but is rarely used in veterinary dentistry. Silver amalgam is a long-standing, excellent restorative material. It has several disadvantages and two advantages in veterinary dentistry. Silver alloy has superior crushing strength over composite filling material and is the filling material of choice for retrograde endodontic therapy. However, its color is a disadvantage as is the cost of additional equipment for its use. Silver amalgam is also more difficult to place properly. Although it can be used to laminate or restore enamel hypoplasia, one of the most

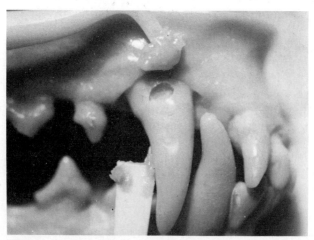

Figure 17. Composite mix is placed into cavity preparation with a plastic filling instrument.

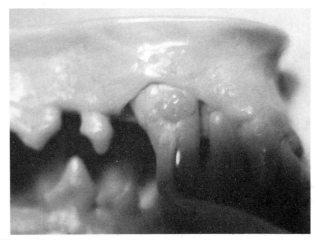

Figure 18. The cavity is overfilled and the composite is allowed to set.

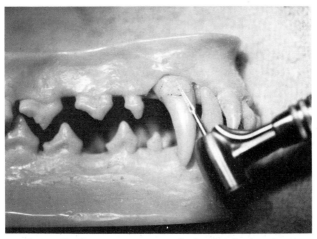

Figure 19. The composite is smoothed with a finishing bur.

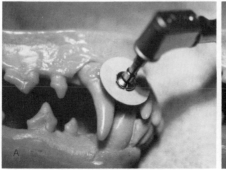
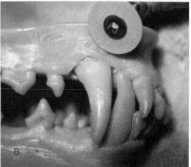

Figure 20. A and B, A sandpaper disk puts a final finish on the composite filling.

common problems in veterinary dentistry, it is esthetically unpleasant and requires additional tooth reduction for retention, thereby weakening an already weak tooth.

Silver alloy comes in zinc and non-zinc forms. The non-zinc form is the choice for retrograde restorations (apical end root canal filling) because it is unaffected by moisture and conditions encountered in retrograde endodontics. The moisture will not affect the setting time or the expansion of the non-zinc alloy. The alloy of choice for restorative dentistry is an alloy containing zinc in a fine-texture form for smoothness of carving, speed of hardening (due to more surface area exposed to mercury), higher copper content to resist corrosion (by resisting the time mercury phase), and ease of polishing. There are many of these "dispersed-phase" alloys available. Type and manufacturer are a matter of choice for the practitioner.

Silver alloy comes in bulk, precapsulated, and pellet forms. The pellet form (Unitek,* for example) is the best for ease of dispersion with the use of a mercury and alloy dispenser. The mercury-alloy mixture is dispensed into a capsule with a mixing pestle inside and placed into an alloy mixing machine called an amalgamator. The amalgamator breaks and mixes the pellet and mercury in 9 to 20 seconds, depending upon the amount of alloy to be mixed (that is, one pellet of alloy and one drop of mercury take about 9 seconds to mix). The silver in pellet or powder bulk form can also be mixed by hand with the use of an amalgam mortar and pestle. This is the least expensive way to mix amalgam. The mixture is simply ground to the desired consistency with the pestle. The precapsulated form, the easiest to use, has the silver and mercury prepackaged in capsule

*Unitek, Monrovia, California.

form. The capsules need only to be placed into the amalgamator and mixed.

The mixed alloy is placed into a dappen dish, carried to the cavity preparation via a silver alloy or amalgam carrier, extruded into the cavity preparation, and condensed thoroughly against the lateral walls and floor of the preparation with an alloy hand condenser or plugger. This is repeated until the cavity is filled. The excess is carved to the original anatomic shape of the tooth with the use of an amalgam carver.

BONDING TECHNIQUE

The restoration of an eroded or hypoplastic enamel surface is best accomplished by an enamel bonding technique and preferably the use of a light-cured composite system, although a chemical-cured composite can be used.

The entire area to be restored is first thoroughly cleaned or pumiced with a plain, nonfluoride, flour pumice (make a thick paste of pumice and water). This is done with a prophylactic handpiece and rubber prophy cup in a slow-speed handpiece.

The pumiced area is thoroughly irrigated with water and dried with an air syringe or canned air (Dust-Off*). It is very important to keep the tooth surface free of salivary contamination. Saliva from the mouth or residual contaminated moisture in the air supply will contaminate the tooth and cause reverse effects of the acid etching process and the bond will fail.

There are many types of acid etch. They come in gel, paste, or liquid forms. These forms vary with manufacturer and all are effective. As with the chemical-cured composite, follow the manufacturer's instructions completely for optimum results. An etching solution (phosphoric acid) is brushed over the defect and surrounding sound enamel for 1 to 2 minutes. Do not allow the etchant to dry or it may become incomplete. The etch is removed with copious amounts of water and thoroughly clean-air dried. Properly etched and dried enamel has a white, frosty appearance. If this is not apparent, re-etch, rinse, and dry. Accidentally etched teeth are remineralized within 1 to 2 days after contamination by the salivary salts.

Unfilled resin or bonding (either light-cured or chemical-cured, depending upon the type of composite to be used) is placed over the area to be restored with a small camel-hair–type brush. Excess resin is removed with air. If a light-cured system is used, the unfilled resin is light-cured at this time before the composite is placed.

*Falcon, Mountainside, New Jersey.

Composite, either chemical-cured or light-cured, is placed over the area to be restored with a plastic instrument in amounts necessary to cover the entire defect and restore the proper anatomic contours of the original tooth. The use of a clean mylar strip to serve as a matrix is, in many cases, advantageous to help establish proper anatomy and to compress the composite over the restoration site. The mylar strip could be used on a canine tooth by wrapping the strip over the composite and around the tooth before curing (Fig. 21).

After curing, the excess composite is trimmed with finishing burs, 8- to 20-sided fluted burs, finishing diamond burs, and sandpaper disks and mandrel in a slow-speed dental handpiece and contra-angle.

After restoring the tooth, the occlusion or bite is checked to make sure there is no interference from opposing teeth when the mouth is closed. If an interference is found, it is relieved until there is no interference or abnormal contact that would fracture the restoration or composite when the animal is awake or chewing.

PIN RETENTION

The use of pins for the retention of filling materials to replace lost tooth structure has limited use in veterinary dentistry. The need

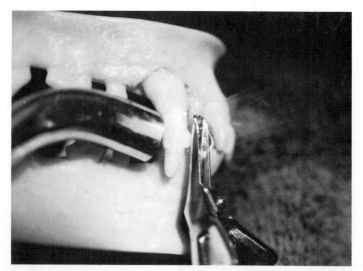

Figure 21. A mylar strip placed around the canine tooth helps to compress the composite into the restoration site.

to build up a tooth to ideal anatomy with silver alloy or composite usually is not needed and rarely succeeds for any length of time owing to the tremendous biting forces placed upon materials designed for the smaller biting forces of man (1200 pounds per square inch in dogs compared with 150 pounds per square inch in man). A show dog should not have added tooth structure or crowns placed in the mouth, for, at this writing, the rules of the American Kennel Club state that a tooth cannot be altered in any way. Therefore, if a crown is fractured or a cusp tip is lost and root canal therapy is needed, the tooth is treated endodontically, simple restoration is placed over the root canal entrance, and the rough edges are removed. No additional tooth height is needed for function.

Pins and posts are needed to build a substructure of tooth for the placement of a crown over the base build-up to give the crown added surface area for retention and support. A brief description of pins is given to familiarize the practitioner with their use should need occur.

Pins are placed within dentin most often in vital teeth; therefore, they must be sufficiently small so as to neither encroach upon the pulp, nor to come too close to the external tooth surface. The veterinarian should give consideration to cavity preparation, tooth morphology, thickness of the remaining dentin, and the location of the pin channel in order to avoid perforation into the pulp or the periodontium.[5] In relating the morphology of the teeth to pin-channel placement,[10] a point midway between the pulp and the external surface of the tooth is assumed to be correct. Canines and premolars usually have enough dentition area for pin placement, but rostral and caudal areas are often marginal. Once the channel location is decided upon, it should be made parallel with the external surface of the tooth rather than its long axis. It is suggested that the operator use only one pin per missing cusp of the tooth and that, where possible, this pin be placed in the area of the line angles. Retention is further increased if the pins are not parallel. Optimal length of the pin into the restorative material is 2 mm; in the dentin, it is is 2 to 3 mm for those retained by dentinal elasticity.[3]

The self-threading pin systems consist of pins that are threaded into undersized channels. The following sizes are available and are listed together with the recommended twist drills for channel preparation: 8 TMS Regular*—0.031 inch pin, 0.027 inch drill; TMS Minim*—0.024 inch pin, 0.021 inch drill; and TMS Minikin*—0.021 inch pin, 0.017 inch drill.[6]

Technique

These channels for pins are placed with drills in a slow-speed handpiece and of a latch-type design. After selection of pin sites, a

---

*Whaledent International, New York, New York.

drill of proper size (that is, a .027 drill for a .031 pin, or a .017 drill for a .021 pin) is placed into the slow-speed handpiece and a channel is drilled into the dentin to the desired 2-mm depth and removed, again paying attention to the relationship of the pulp to the channel to be drilled and the external surface of the tooth.[5] Channels should be at least 0.5 mm from the dentinoenamel junction.[10] The proper-sized pin is either placed into the latch-type slow-speed handpiece and threaded into the channel or the pins can be obtained in the hand-threaded design and threaded into the channel by hand with the use of a hand chuck provided by manufacturers (Figs. 22 and 23). Whaledent International has an excellent procedure guide for the use of thread-mate pins. The restorative material is applied over the pins and finished as previously described.

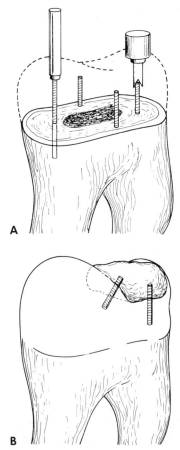

Figure 22. Placement of self-threading pins to aid in retention of restorative material. *A*, Self-threading pin system (retained by dentinal elasticity) placed in a fourth premolar to show the direction of the drill channel, the distance from the pulpal wall, depth of pin placement necessary for retention, and use of hand chuck for pin placement. *B*, Pins to aid in the retention of restorative material. *Note*: Added occlusal height is unnecessary. Restorative material should only extend to height of remaining tooth structure.

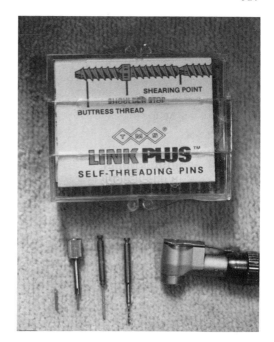

Figure 23. Self-threading pins. *Left* to *right*, Hand-threaded pin, pin with hand chuck, pin in latch-type attachment, twisted drill, and low-speed handpiece.

PULP TREATMENTS

Often deep carious lesions or fracture sites encroach upon the pulp chamber with or without exposing it. The pulp chamber or canal must be protected from the external environment and from encroachment of the filling material and their pulpal irritation to prevent pulpal necrosis and eventual abcessation. Presently available pulp-treatment materials may be classified into (1) cavity washes and medicaments; (2) cavity varnishes; (3) liners; and (4) bases. The literature is replete with studies pertaining to the properties and uses of available materials. It is imperative that the practitioner be aware of the types of materials available for use and that he or she understands the effects these materials have on the dental pulp.

Cavity varnishes are solutions of an organic solvent and resins. Their main function is to act as a seal and prevent microleakage around the margins of restorations into dentinal tubules.[11] Varnishes reduce, but do not entirely prevent, penetration of acids from overlying cements into the dentinal tubules. They are regarded as being relatively ineffective in reducing thermal conductivity.[12] Varnishes should not be used under composite resin restorations because the organic solvent in the varnish may enter into the setting reaction of the resin material. The varnishes are applied with a cotton pledget dipped in solution and placed in and around the cavity preparation and air-dried.

Cavity liners should be reserved for extremely thin film dispersions of calcium hydroxide or zinc oxide-eugenol applied to one or more cavity walls in the proximity of the pulp. These liners are suspensions of calcium hydroxide or zinc oxide-eugenol in either a volatile organic liquid or in an aqueous solution. Following application, their solvents quickly evaporate, leaving a thin film of residue, which is insufficient to provide a good thermal barrier. As the sole protecting medium in deep cavity preparations, cavity liners are inadequate. They should be overlaid with an appropriate base. Calcium hydroxide is the indicated material of choice as the initial lining medium for direct pulp capping procedures. It has the capability of inducing reparative dentin deposition but does not have an obtundent effect on the pulp. Because of its low compressive strength, calcium hydroxide should be overlaid with a stronger basing medium, such as reinforced zinc oxide-eugenol or zinc phosphate cement, before placement of a final restoration. Zinc oxide-eugenol probably has been used more for pulp protection and sedation than any other agent. It is considered an obtundent capable of soothing a traumatized or slightly inflamed pulp.[11] In deep cavity preparation with no pulp exposure, reinforced zinc oxide-eugenol is an excellent intermediary basing medium. However, in cases in which pulp exposures are definite or suspected, a liner of calcium hydroxide should precede the use of zinc oxide-eugenol. The calcium hydroxide powder mixed with sterile water is placed over the cavity wall and air-dried. The zinc oxide-eugenol is placed over the calcium hydroxide and the excess is removed from cavity walls.

Among the materials available for basing are the polycarboxylate cements[14] and the reinforced zinc oxide-eugenol cements. Reinforced zinc oxide-eugenol cements possess greater compressive strength than the regular zinc oxide-eugenol cements. They are mixed per manufacturers' instructions and placed over the pulpal walls. The thickness of dentin remaining between the cutting instrument and the pulp is an important consideration. Two millimeters of remaining dentin is indicated as a safety dimension for the pulp, providing adequate protection from the trauma of cavity preparation. As this dimension is reduced, pulpal response increases proportionately.

Indirect Pulp Capping

The treatment of an area of vital pulp tissue with the hope that the recuperative power of the remaining pulp is sufficient to restore it to health is referrred to as pulp capping. When the medicaments used are applied to the pulp indirectly through a small amount of carious dentin left over a suspected pulp exposure, the procedure is referred to as indirect pulp capping. The carious process is hopefully arrested and the pulp stimulated to form a barrier of reparative dentin. It is further desired that remineralization of the partially decalcified dentin will take place.[14]

Treatment materials used in indirect pulp capping differ little from those used in deep cavity preparations from which all caries have been removed. Cavity washes, medicaments, cavity liners, and bases are used as previously described.[5]

Direct Pulp Capping

Calcium hydroxide is the material of choice in the treatment of exposed pulp tissue. If it is used in a cavity liner form, it should be overlaid with a pressureless, thin layer of zinc oxide-eugenol and then followed by a high compressive strength cement mixed to a base consistency. This will prevent possible intrusion of the weaker underlying cavity liner into the pulp.

The clinician should make every effort to place the properly indicated restoration in the tooth as soon as possible after the application of the pulpal treatment materials. This will help prevent gross contamination of the dressing and/or healing site by the oral fluids. In addition, the final restoration should exhibit good marginal sealing properties and withstand the rigors of the oral environment for an extended period of time.[5]

REFERENCES

1. Bell, B. H., and Gainger, D. A.: Nomenclature and armamentarium. Basic Op. Dent. Proc., 20:5–17, 1971.
2. Caputo, A. A., and Standlee, J. P.: Pins and posts: Why, when, and how. Dental Clin. North Am., 20:299–307, 1976.
3. Caputo, A. A., Standlee, J. P., and Collard, E. W.: The mechanics of load transfer by retentive pins. J. Pros. Dent., 29:442–449, 1973.
4. Colley, I. T., Hampson, E. L., and Lehman, M. L.: Retention of post crowns. Br. Dent. J., 124:63–69, 1968.
5. Dilts, W. E., and Coury, T. L.: A conservative approach to the placement of retentive pins. Dental Clin. North Am., 20:397–402, 1976.
6. Hanson, E. C., and Caputo, A. A.: Cementing mediums and retentive characteristics of dowels. J. Pros. Dent., 32:551–557, 1974.
7. Kinzer, R. L., and Morris, C.: Instruments and instrumentation to promote conservative operative dentistry. Dental Clin. North Am., 20:290–296, 1976.
8. Mendel, R. W.: Indirect pulp capping: Some whys, whens, and hows. J. Kentucky Dent. Assoc., 26:22–27, 1974.
9. Miranda, F. J., Collard, E. W., and Hatch, R. A.: Diagnosis and treatment of pulpal distress. Dental Clin. North Am., 20:290–296, 1976.
10. Moffa, J. P., Razzano, M. R., and Doyle, M. G.: Pins: A comparison of their retentive properties. J. Am. Dental Assoc., 78:5229–5235, 1969.
11. Mostzeller, J. H.: The ability of a prednisolone solution to eliminate pulpal inflammation. J. Pros. Dent., 13:754–760, 1963.
12. Stanley, H. R.: Pulpal response to dental techniques and materials. Dental Clin. North Am., 15:115–126, 1971.

13. Swerdlow, H., Stanley, H. R., and Sayegh, F. S.: Minimizing pulpal reactions with prednisone therapy, J. Oral Ther. Pharmacol., *1*:593–601, 1965.
14. Trulove, E. L., Mitchell, D. F., and Phillips, R. W.: Biological evaluation of carboxylate cement. J. Dent. Res., *50*:166, 1971.
15. Welk, D. A., and Laswell, H. A.: Rationale for designing cavity preparations in light of current knowledge and technology. Dental Clin. North Am., *20*:238–239, 1976.

Animal Dentistry
College of Veterinary Medicine and Biomedical Sciences
Colorado State University
Fort Collins, Colorado 80523

0195–5616/86 $0.00 + .20

Restorative Dentistry

Clinical Applications

*Charles A. Williams, D.V.M.**

In veterinary practice, the most common indications for tooth restoration are as follows:

1. Fillings for teeth damaged by caries or those with drill sites as access for endodontic therapy.
2. Enamel hypoplasia.
3. Chipped or fractured crowns.

The use of silver amalgam and composite resins for the placement of fillings has already been described in this publication. "Systems other than the acrylic resins or its derivatives have been synthesized and studied. These include polycarboxylate, epoxy, cyanoacrylate, and polyester resins. Theoretically, each has certain advantages but invariably they have proved unsuccessful because of other deficiencies."[4] An excellent review of the literature in the field has been published.[3]

Cavity preparation and filling have been well described in the article "Restorative Dentistry." This article will consist of a pictorial case presentation describing various types of crown restorations.

ENAMEL HYPOPLASIA

The lesions of enamel hypoplasia occur during the development of the permanent teeth. In general, any febrile or generally debilitating disease during the developmental stages may cause lack of proper mineralization of the enamel.[2]

Infections with epitheliotropic viruses, such as the canine distemper virus, are particularly incriminated in the development of enamel hypoplasia; thus, the term "distemper teeth" has been used

*Director, Blue Cross Animal Hospital, Inc., Fairfax, Virginia

to describe this condition. Other possible causes are periapical inflammation or trauma affecting the permanent tooth bud, nutritional deficiencies, and endocrine dysfunction.[1]

Enamel hypoplasia may occur as small, localized lesions recognized as rough, cup-like depressions in the tooth surface of a single tooth or it may be generalized, with incomplete mineralization of all of the teeth.

When all of the teeth are involved, it is not practical to attempt crown restoration. In these cases, it is usually best to smooth and polish the teeth and encourage as much home cleaning as possible. However, when a single tooth or two has localized enamel hypoplasia, the crown can easily be restored to its natural beauty and function by using an acid-etch technique and a composite resin enamel restorative. It should be noted, however, that a crown restored by use of a composite resin is never as strong as the normal enamel; therefore, chewing vices such as cage chewing and rock chewing will easily destroy such a restoration. Owners of these animals should be so advised and cautioned to avoid letting the pet engage in such chewing habits.

In the first case (Fig. 1), the coronal one third of a maxillary canine tooth is missing its normal enamel covering. The tooth is prepared by grinding away the rough, stained, and pitted area feathering out to the normal part of the crown by using a high-speed drill with a pear-shaped bur. The remaining enamel is acid-etched for 2 to 3 minutes. A composite restorative material is applied using plastic instruments or a mylar strip. An alternative way of prepping the tooth in order to achieve maximum retention of the restorative

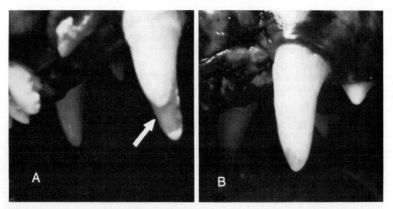

Figure 1. Canine tooth with enamel hypoplasia before (A) and after (B) repair with chemically activated composite material.

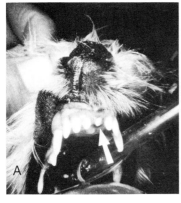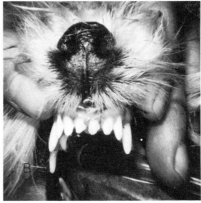

Figure 2. Incisors with enamel hypoplasia before (A) and after (B) repair with photo-activated composite material.

material is to use an inverted cone bur to undercut grooves circular and longitudinal in the dentin core.[3]

In the second case of enamel hypoplasia (Fig. 2), an intermediate maxillary incisor is missing the entire coronal one third of the tooth. Because there has been no pulp exposure in this case, endodontic treatment is not necessary. The remaining part of the crown can be prepped and etched as previously described, and the composite material used to sculpture a new crown. To give additional stability and retention of this type of restoration, the composite can be anchored to the stump by using a pin system (Thread-mate system*). The use of this technique will be demonstrated in subsequent cases.

RESTORATION OF FRACTURED TEETH

If the enamel is chipped from a tooth without exposing the pulp cavity, it can be restored using techniques identical to repair of enamel hypoplasia. On the other hand, once the pulp has been exposed, endodontic treatment must be completed before the crown can be restored. After root canal therapy, the access site can be filled and the crown restored by using the composite resin to sculpture a new tooth (Fig. 3).

This type of repair is quite fragile, however, and can be chipped off with vigorous chewing. An alternative technique that provides

---

*Whaledent International, New York. New York.

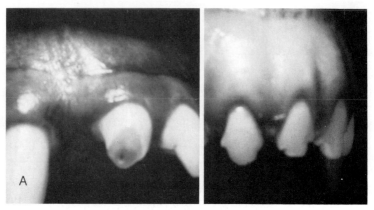

Figure 3. A, Fractured incisor before repair. B, Fractured incisor after root canal and photo-activated composite material.

much greater holding power is the use of pins or posts that are cemented into the dentin of the tooth stump and act as reinforcing rods. This works much like using rebar (iron rods) to support poured concrete in construction work. This technique is indicated anytime an undercut cannot be used and where a substantial amount of crown needs to be built up. The main difference between pins and posts is that posts are generally placed down the pulp canal and pins are placed into holes drilled into the dentin. In the case of a slab fracture of the upper fourth premolar (carnassial tooth), TMS pins can be used to support the composite restorative material (Fig. 4).

The number of pins and the angle at which they are placed depend upon the fractured tooth stump, but, in general, as many pins as possible should be used without substantially weakening the supporting dentin or undermining the remaining enamel. They should be placed at an angle that will best facilitate the sculpturing of the new crown to duplicate the original shape. In molding a new crown, one must be sure to check the occlusion. If the "new" tooth does not fit perfectly, it must be ground down so that no occlusal trauma occurs. When repairing canine teeth, it is often prudent to make the restored tooth slightly shorter than the normal or opposite tooth. In this way, excess trauma and strain on the prosthesis can be reduced. Figure 5 shows a canine tooth that has been restored using TMS pins as described.

In many cases, especially when restoring fractured canine teeth, a heavier post, cemented deep into the stump, makes for a stronger

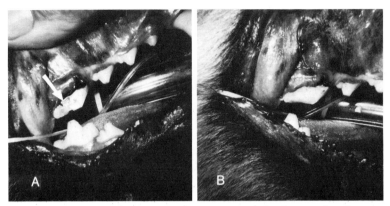

Figure 4. A, Example of fractured upper fourth premolar (carnassial) with TMS pins cemented into the dentin. B, Same tooth after adding composite resin restorative material.

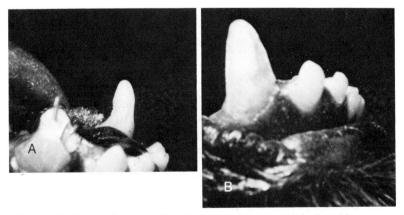

Figure 5. A, Fractured canine tooth with TMS pins. B, Same tooth after adding composite resin restorative material.

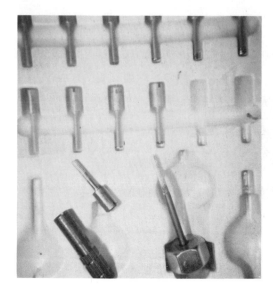

Figure 6. Example of a post kit including a drill and a wrench.

prosthesis than the smaller TMS pins. Post kits come with drills to tap the pulp canal and a wrench to screw the post into place (see Fig. 6). Endodontic treatment prior to the placement of posts is obviously necessary.

In Figure 7, we can see how the pulp canal of a fractured canine tooth is enlarged to accept a gold post. Once the canal is tapped, the post is cemented in place using a carboxylate cement (Durelon,* for example). Allowing a few minutes for the cement to set, the composite material can then be used to mold the new crown. When covering a post with a tooth-shaded composite, it is important to use the proper shade. Most composites developed for restoration of human teeth are a darker shade of yellow than the teeth found in most pet animals. Furthermore, a thin layer of composite over a darker-colored post will refract the color of the post, making the restored crown too dark a shade (Fig. 8).

CAPS

The most sophisticated type of crown restoration is also the strongest and often the most rewarding. It is the metal cap, which must be precisely custom-designed and fitted. Very exacting impres-

---

*Premier Dental Products Co., Norristown, Pennsylvania.

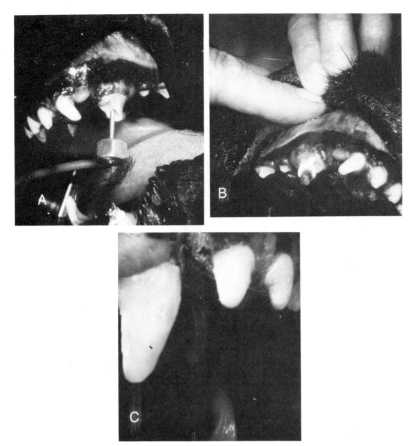

Figure 7. A, Using drill from post kit to tap the pulp canal (a root canal procedure has been performed prior to fitting the post). B, The post is cemented in place. C, The restored tooth after adding a composite resin material.

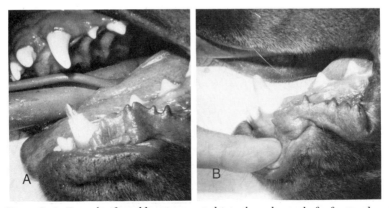

Figure 8. A, Example of a gold post cemented into the pulp canal of a fractured canine tooth. B, Same tooth after adding a composite restorative material. Note that, in this case, the shade of the restorative material is too dark and doesn't match the tooth perfectly.

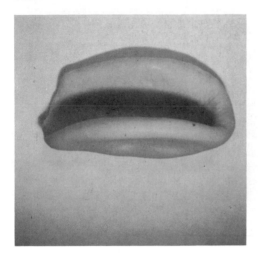

Figure 9. Custom-made tray for use in taking impressions of a fractured canine tooth.

sions must be taken and models made so that a dental lab can design a metal crown that fits perfectly. Because most of the supplies needed to perform this task are designed for humans, even the impression trays must be customized. Plastic trays can be designed using Formatray.*

In customizing a tray, it is important to remember that the tray must be deep enough to go over the entire tooth (or stump) well past the gingival margin. Furthermore, the tray must be made of a nonflexible material so that the impression material within cannot move and distort as the tray is handled. An example of a tray made for the stump of a canine tooth of a dog is shown in Figure 9.

In order to keep the impression material from spilling over the open ends of the tray, clay or weatherstripping material can be used to plug them (Fig. 10). This method will permit the tray to fit over adjacent teeth while still holding the impression material in place.

Rubber-based impression material (Impregum,† for example) must be used in order to get the precise detail necessary for making a cap.

The stump must be prepared by grinding down the remaining enamel by a couple of millimeters at the top and taper to just beneath the gum (Fig. 11). This is to allow the cap to cover the stump without increasing the overall diameter of the restored tooth. Next, gingival retraction cord is placed into the gingival sulcus so that the free gingival margin is held away from the neck of the tooth,

---

*Kerr Division, Sybron Corp., Romulus, Michigan.
†Premier Dental Products, Norristown, Pennsylvania.

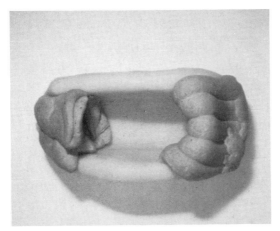

Figure 10. Impression tray with weatherstripping material used to plug the open ends.

thus allowing the impression material to flow into the depth of the sulcus.

The two-part chemically activated impression material is spatulated together. The tray is filled and the material is placed over the tooth stump (Fig. 12), where it is held perfectly still until the impression material hardens (about 2 to 3 minutes). Once the impression material is set up, it is removed with one brisk pull, snapping it away from the tooth.

When a custom post is to be made, it is important to be sure that the pulp canal has been sufficiently widened at the top and

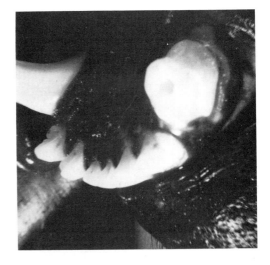

Figure 11. Fractured canine tooth that has been prepared for a custom-made crown and is ready to have impressions taken.

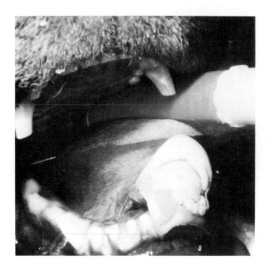

Figure 12. Custom-made impression tray filled with rubber-base impression material being placed over the fractured tooth that has been prepared for receiving a crown.

tapered in funnel fashion so that the impression material will come out. If it is accidently undercut (that is, wider within the tooth than at the opening), the impression material will be retained.

Alginate impressions must also be taken of both the upper and lower arches (Fig. 13). An occlusal impression is also needed. The occlusal impression can be taken by mixing a batch of alginate, then placing a wad of the material in the palm of the hand. The

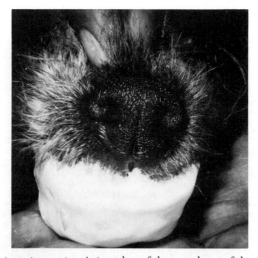

Figure 13. Alginate impressions being taken of the rostral part of the upper dental arch of a dog.

anesthetized patient is then made to bite down into the alginate wad for about 60 seconds as the material sets up.

Pink stone models are made from the alginate impressions (Fig. 14). These plus the occlusal impression and the rubber base impression of the broken tooth stump are sent to a dental lab. The lab is instructed as to how you wish to have the post and crown custom-made. Usually they can duplicate the corresponding normal tooth on the opposite side. The tooth stump is then given a temporary filling (Fig. 15), and the patient is sent home until the cap can be made.

The lab time for this procedure averages about 1 week. When the cap is designed, the models will be put on an articulator so that the occlusal pattern can be simulated (Fig. 16). This enables the lab to customize the crown so that it will fit perfectly with no occlusal trauma. A custom post can be designed to give added stability. When possible, a mushroom-like design allows the post to envelope the tip of the stump and the dowel to fit into the core of the tooth (Fig. 17). This gives it even greater holding power.

When the time comes to install the prosthesis, the temporary filling is drilled away (Fig. 18). First the post is cemented in place with carboxylate cement (Fig. 19), then the metal cap is installed, again held firm with carboxylate cement (Fig. 20). This makes a very substantial repair that will not fracture. However, very aggressive dogs can still rip the prosthetic crown off the stump if enough force is applied. In patients known to abuse themselves this way, an additional technique to add stability is recommended. Cross pins can be placed through the metal cap perpendicular to the surface of the crown and cemented deep into the dentin of the stump (Fig. 21). This will provide the ultimate in holding power and will ensure the retention of the cap in all but the most difficult patients.

Text continued on page 937

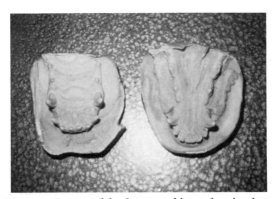

Figure 14. Stone models of upper and lower dental arches.

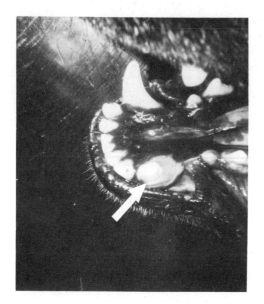

Figure 15. A temporary filling is placed in the fractured tooth, which has been prepared for a custom-made post and crown.

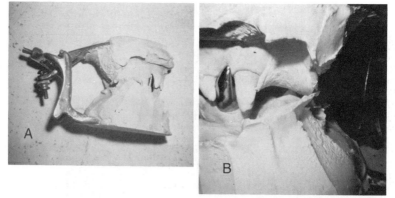

Figure 16. A, Stone models with custom-made metal crown on an articulation. B, Close-up of metal crown on stone model showing perfect occlusal fit.

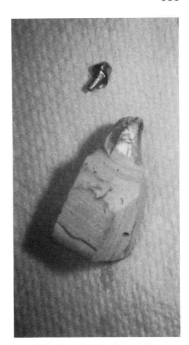

Figure 17. Custom-made post next to stone model of the fractured tooth.

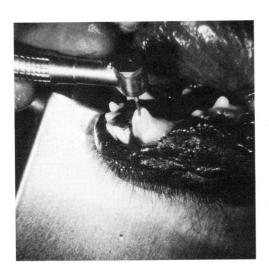

Figure 18. The temporary filling is drilled away.

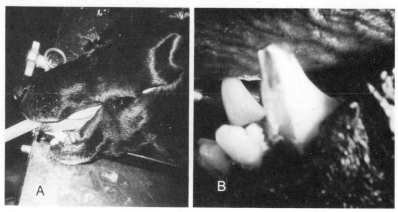

Figure 19. *A*, Metal post is cemented into fractured canine tooth. *B*, Close-up showing perfect fit.

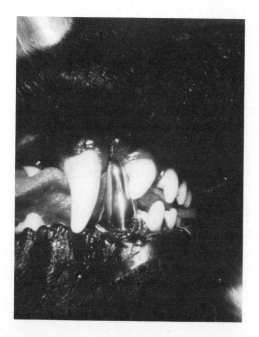

Figure 20. Metal crown that has been cemented over the post inserted into stump of a fractured canine tooth.

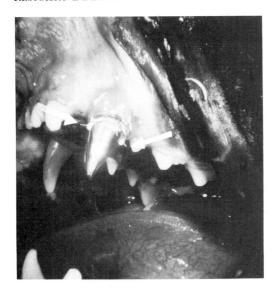

Figure 21. Example of cross-pinning to add greater rotational stability to metal crown.

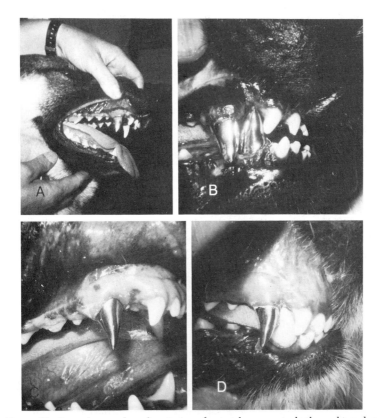

Figure 22. Several examples of custom-made metal crowns in both working dogs and pets.

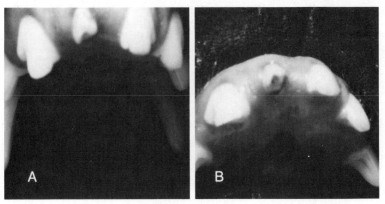

Figure 23. A and B, Two views of a fractured incisor that has been prepped to receive a crown.

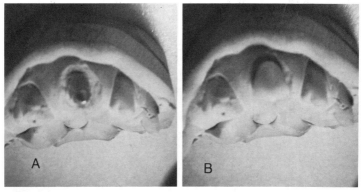

Figure 24. A, Custom-made post on stone model. B, Custom-made porcelain crown on stone model.

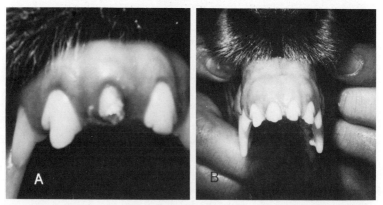

Figure 25. A, Metal post cemented into the stump of a fractured incisor. B, Porcelain crown restoration of fractured incisor.

Metal crowns have been used in all breeds and types of dogs. Although the biggest demand for metal crowns may be seen in police, military, or guard dogs, these prosthetic teeth work efficiently for working breeds and household pets as well (Fig. 22).

The all-metal crowns are probably the most durable and trouble-free; however, the stainless-steel look may be objectional to some owners. When this is the case, a porcelain crown can be made. These tooth-shaded look-alikes do have a nice cosmetic appearance, but bad chewing habits will chip these crowns and may necessitate replacement. Nevertheless, they do make a beautiful repair, especially for the teeth that are not likely to take a great deal of abuse.

Figure 23 shows the mouth of a Collie dog with an accidental fracture of a maxillary central incisor. The technique previously described was used to make a custom post and crown (Fig. 24). The prosthesis was cemented into place using carboxylate cement, with beautiful cosmetic and functional results (Fig. 25).

SUMMARY

Restorative techniques for human teeth have been used and refined for centuries. Most of these techniques can be applied with few modifications to restore diseased or damaged teeth in animals. The results can be both functionally sound and cosmetically pleasing.

REFERENCES

1. Harvey, C.: Veterinary Dentistry. Philadelphia, W. B. Saunders Co., 1985, p. 81.
2. Eisenmenger, E., and Zetner, K.: Veterinary Dentistry. Philadelphia, Lea & Febiger, 1985, pp. 58–61.
3. Paffenbarger, G. C.: Dental Cements, Direct Filling Resins, Composite and Adhesive Restorative Materials: A Resume. Journal of Biomedical Material Research. No. 2, Part 2, 1972, p. 363.
4. Phillips, R. W.: Restorative resins. Dent. Clin. North Am., 19(2):233, 1975.

Blue Cross Animal Hospital, Inc.
8429 Lee Highway
Fairfax, Virginia 22031

Dentistry   0195–5616/86 $0.00 + .20

Orthodontics for the Dog

Treatment Methods

Donald L. Ross, D.V.M., M.S.*

PREVENTING ORTHODONTIC PROBLEMS

The prevention of orthodontic problems is centered in two areas. The control of genetically induced problems by careful selection of individuals without oral defects for breeding and the elimination of those problems induced by the deciduous teeth. The reduction of genetic abnormalities will require the expansion of the oral description as given in the breed standards. When breed enthusiasts and judges have an adequate understanding of oral structure, the ability to improve is enhanced. The description of correct occlusion, accompanied by a uniform method of grading dentition, must come from veterinarians knowledgeable in the area. The second area, deciduous teeth, can be considered from the basis of the genetic involvement in the retention of deciduous teeth and from the mechanical effects of deciduous retention on other oral structures. There is little doubt that there is a strong genetic basis for the retention of deciduous teeth. The characteristic has not been fully defined in terms of type of genetic pattern involved. The emphasis has been on the prevention of problems created by the mechanical presence of the deciduous teeth. However, the selection of breeding stock in which the deciduous teeth are shed at the proper time certainly reduces the problems seen in the occlusion. When retention of deciduous teeth is known to be a problem in a given line of breeding, the advantage of early extraction becomes obvious. Many of the common orthodontic problems can be prevented if they are detected in time. When considering the mechanical effects of retention, it must be realized that not only must a

*Veterinary Dental Clinic, Houston, Texas

tooth fall out at the proper time but the root resorption that allows the exfoliation must begin at the proper time in relation to the developing permanent teeth. The root structure of deciduous teeth forms rapidly after the eruption of the crown and almost as rapidly begins the resorption process to make room for the permanent tooth. When the resorption is delayed, the permanent tooth bud is forced to alter its normal eruptive pathway and, once diverted, may never regain normal position. When the deciduous teeth erupt in an incorrect relationship, the force of the interlocking action against the opposite arch is enough to alter growth patterns that would otherwise be dictated by genetics.

When the deciduous occlusion is abnormal, extraction allows the development of the mouth to take place under the influence of genetics alone. Early extraction of deciduous teeth, at 6 to 8 weeks of age, often allows what would have become a severe prognathic or brachygnathic defect to correct by the time the permanent teeth erupt. As a rule of thumb, extract the teeth from the shorter jaw that would block the forward growth of that jaw. Extraction of teeth involved in blocking jaw growth may be effective as late as the twelfth week, even though there will be only 2 or 3 weeks before the permanent teeth begin to erupt. The extraction does nothing to stimulate jaw growth; it just removes a mechanical barrier to the expression of genetic growth potential.

The extraction of deciduous teeth should be approached with care and a knowledge of the biology of mouth development in mind. Damage of the single-cell thick layer of epithelial tissue that forms enamel is possible if the deciduous tooth is extracted carelessly. If the extraction is done carelessly in the early stages of development of the permanent teeth, damage to the enamel-forming tissue of the permanent teeth is a real possibility. This usually occurs when the elevator is pushed too deeply into the alveolar socket of the deciduous tooth. Another frequent mistake in the removal of deciduous teeth is allowing the root structure to remain following root fracture. The remaining root structure may or may not be rapidly resorbed by the body. When the root tip remains, it continues to occupy space and alter the path of eruption of the permanent tooth. The possibility of infection exists, although the incidence is usually low. It is not uncommon to see broken deciduous root tips persist for several months before being resorbed or expelled from the alveolar bone by abcessation.

OCCLUSAL ADJUSTMENTS

The marked resistance of the canine and feline teeth to bacterial decay makes occlusal adjustments a useful technique. The most common application is in the incisal area when a lack of arch length results in crowding and/or rotation of the teeth. A safe-sided diamond disk is used to remove small amounts of tooth substance from both the mesial and distal surfaces of all six incisors. It is better to remove a small amount of material from all six incisors rather than a larger area from only two or three teeth. The disk is used until it can be passed between the contacting surface of the teeth. The available space can then be used to allow incisors to assume the correct position.

Altering the form of the lower canine is necessary in some palatal fractures. The midline palatal fracture often allows a slight posterior, but stable, shift of one side of the maxilla and creates an occlusal interference between the maxillary and mandibular canines. The reduction of length and possibly adding a reverse bevel to the contacting tips of the canines will frequently eliminate the occlusal interference.

SIMPLE TOOTH MOVEMENTS

Simple tooth movements are most often considered to be the movement of a single tooth in a single direction. The orthodontic problems seen most frequently in the dog offer several examples of simple tooth movement. With the maxillary canine, rostral displacement occurs when the root structure of the deciduous canine fails to resorb or resorbs too slowly. The mandibular canine erupts lingually and sometimes rostrally. With either rostral or lingual displacement of the lower canine, there is almost always rostral movement of the lower incisors. Other examples include the lingual shift of the maxillary fourth premolar, most often seen in Shelties and Collies, and the lateral eruption of the maxillary lateral incisor.

Techniques used in correction of these abnormalities are quite varied. The caudal movement of the maxillary canine may be accomplished by either constructing a removable maxillary acrylic plate or using the maxillary fourth premolar/first molar as anchorage for elastics to the canine. If the acrylic plate is used (see the descriptions of basic acrylic units), the lingual post of the affected canine is replaced by a trailing arm for the attachment of elastics to the canine. A 0.03 to 0.036 wire is formed to lie along the lingual base of the premolars and exit between the second and third premolar to form a hook on the buccal surface. The advantage of the acrylic lies in the daily removal for cleaning and lack of soft-tissue damage. If the posterior teeth are used for anchorage, a sublingual wire is placed in a figure-eight around the two teeth, with the point of twist at the rostrobuccal edge of the fourth premolar. The twist is formed into a loop, with the free end on the gingival side of the loop. An elastic of appropriate length and strength is fitted into the loop and stretched forward over the canine. A bracket on the buccal surface of the canine is needed to stop the movement of the elastic up and down the tooth surface. The disadvantages of this technique involve the soft-tissue destruction in the sublingual area on the anchor tooth.

Lingual displacements of the mandibular canine are corrected with a palatal acrylic plate. The acrylic unit functions as a bite plane, with the displaced canine(s) contacting the acrylic before the teeth close into their normal rest position. The build-up of acrylic necessary at the contact point of the lower canine may be shaped so that slight rostral or caudal movement of the lower canine is achieved along with the lateral movement of the tooth. The units may take as little as 5 to 10 days to move the lower canine in the 6- to 10-month-old dog or up to 3 to 5 weeks in the older animal. The unit can usually be discarded when movement is complete. A retainer device is normally not needed. In the younger animals, the mandibular canine must at least contact the maxillary soft tissue before the correcting unit is put in place and often it is desirable to wait until the rapid spurt in head growth that accompanies eruption of the permanent teeth is past. This may mean allowing the mandibular canine to create some soft-tissue damage in the 5- to 7-month age range but this is better than having the acrylic unit restrict the growth of the maxilla during this period of life. If possible, do not wait until the pressure on the mandibular canine created by contact with the maxilla suppresses the eruption of the lower canine. If the oral eruption is interrupted, the root structure continues to form but pushes its way distally into the mandible. This type of growth results in a shorter clinical crown and a visible size discrepancy when compared with the other mandibular canine. In the mature animal, this effect may be multiplied in the lateral tilting of the tooth, which results in additional loss of height. If the height loss is sufficient, the tooth may not have enough contact with the buccal surface of the maxilla to hold it in its new position after the appliance is removed. Increase in clinical crown height may be achieved with other appliance forms but is more difficult when working with the extremely large root structure of the canine teeth.

Movement of lateral incisors that have extra space between the incisor and the rest of the incisor group can be either relatively simple or complex enough to require two or three appliance types to accomplish the movement. If the lateral incisor is just spaced too far away from the others, elastic retraction is usually quick and easy. The other five incisors are used as anchorage by placing brackets on the adjacent intermediate incisor and opposite lateral incisor and using an arch bar as an attachment device for an elastic to the malpositioned lateral incisor. The arch bar and incisal arch are stabilized by using direct bond composite restorative material at the contact point of the arch bar with each of the incisors. The position of the bracket on the affected lateral incisor is critical to achieve the desired movement and alignment with the others as the space is closed.

More frequently, the laterally displaced corner incisor also is rotationally out of position and may even be tilted dorsally as well as laterally. In these cases, more than one appliance may be required to accomplish correct position. The dorsal tipping and rotational abnormalities should be corrected before attempting to totally close the space between it and the adjacent intermediate incisor.

ROTATIONAL TECHNIQUES

The most frequently encountered rotational displacements are seen in the premolar portion of the maxillary arch. Unfortunately, these teeth rotate because of a lack of arch length when compared with the width of the teeth that have to occupy the space. To consider correction of these rotational problems necessitates the rostral or caudal movement of the adjacent teeth (which is usually difficult or impossible) or the extraction of one or more of the smaller premolars to make room for the rotated second or third premolar. Extraction is often unacceptable for those animals in conformation competition, but if extraction is acceptable to the owner, it is obviously easier and quicker to extract the rotated teeth to improve the periodontal health than to go through the orthodontic procedures. Thus, the actual number of situations in which rotation of a premolar is necessary is quite small.

The same basic principle applies to rotational abnormalities in the incisal area. They occur because of a lack of arch space in comparison with total tooth width. Extraction of the rotated incisors is the quickest way to periodontal health. The notable exception to this is the case in which the rostral/lingual eruption of the mandibular canine reduces the arch space available for the lower incisors. The spreading of the lower canines with a palatal bite plane usually creates enough space for proper incisal alignment. When the canine pressure is relieved, the incisors will often realign without orthodontic intervention if given a few months time.

TIPPING PROBLEMS

By definition, tipping is the movement of the crown without changing the position of the root apex. In practice, many treatment techniques result in tipping because of the inability to properly adapt human materials to animal anatomy. This form of orthodontic movement is the easiest and quickest to accomplish but also is the most likely to result in structural damage. This is particularly true when the direction of movement is in a facial or buccal direction.

Clinically, the problems usually approached with tipping techniques include the facial drift of the mandibular central incisors, the lingual displacement of incisors resulting from crowding, and the lateral movement of mandibular canines. The mandibular centrals that drift forward present a particular problem in that the drifting process is the result of inadequate osseous support. Radiographically, almost all of these cases show an increase in the width of the mandibular symphysis and a decrease in the density of the alveolar bone around the roots of these teeth. Within a few weeks after the treatment is completed, the teeth will drift back to their original position because of the lack of osseous support.

The appliance design for the movement of mandibular canines has been described previously. The movement of the mandibular centrals is usually accomplished with elastic ligature thread. Brackets are positioned on the mandibular central and lateral incisors; occasionally, brackets are needed on the lower canines to help maintain elastic position. The elastic thread is applied so that it encircles the lower canine and incisors, then the segment of thread going across the floor of the mouth is brought forward to the lingual (back) surface of the lower centrals. If the tooth is too small for a bracket, the elastic may be attached to the teeth using a ligature wire around each tooth, with the twist on the lingual side, and forming the wire twist into a loop to receive the elastic thread. A thin acrylic plate across the floor of the mouth may be necessary to keep the elastic from cutting into the tissue during tooth movement. If it is needed, it is usually adequately stabilized by the elastic. Be sure to cut out enough space to allow the incisors to move to the desired position, but closely adapt the plate to the lingual contour of the other teeth.

The forward movement of crowded and lingually displaced incisors can be accomplished by adding a removable acrylic plate and a microscrew behind the teeth to be moved. The microscrew can then be adjusted every other day to gradually effect the forward movement of the incisors.

BODY MOVEMENTS

The rostral/caudal movements of teeth are preferably accomplished as body movements—that is, the root of the tooth is moved along the same plane as the crown. This results in a much more stable tooth when the movement is complete, because the pressures applied to the tooth in daily activities are absorbed along the natural planes of oral structure. This is contrasted to tipping techniques, in which the relationship of the crown to the root and bone structure is altered. In the dog, these body movements are technically harder to achieve. They require the use of orthodontic brackets and "square" wire. The wire precisely fits the slot in the bracket, and the forces are transmitted to the tooth in a manner that does not allow tipping of the crown.

The utilization of these techniques requires an in-depth understanding of forming arch wire, including stepping techniques, tipping bends, opening and closing loops, and so forth. This is beyond the scope of this discussion, however.

ADJUSTING THE CROWN HEIGHT

Adjusting the height of the crown of a tooth involves movement of the root structure either into or out of the alveolar socket. Because this movement is more in opposition to the periodontal ligament fibers than to the alveolar bone, the movement must be slower and precisely controlled. If the forces exceed the rate of periodontal ligament fiber adjustment, the destruction of these fibers results in rapid loosening of the tooth and even extraction of the tooth. There are many instances in which the crown height is out of alignment with adjacent teeth. The delayed eruption or impaction of teeth, crowding of teeth, and sometimes poorly planned orthodontic therapy produce the problem.

Two major types of appliances are used to elevate or depress the tooth. The choice depends on the tooth involved and the amount of movement needed. In the incisal area, either a segmental arch wire or an acrylic plate with a spring positioned to effect the desired movement may be used. An incisal arch wire is most effective when dealing with the centrals or intermediates. Brackets are positioned on all incisors and a wire bent to passively rest in the brackets at the desired position of the teeth. The wire is then forced into the bracket of the tooth to be moved, and the pressure of the arch wire effects the movement. If the needed movement is more than a millimeter, it is better to effect movement in stages, by rebending the arch wire as the tooth moves. The segmental arch wire is difficult to utilize in the smaller breeds because of the difficulty in cementing the large human orthodontic brackets.

The acrylic plate with a spring-lever arm can be used on any tooth in the mouth. Its versatility lies in the multitude of wire sizes and shapes that can be designed to effect movement. The lever arm can be designed to effect movement in more than one direction. The lever arm can be activated in degrees to reduce the stress on the tooth at any given time. Most units can be used as removable appliances.

ADVANCED TECHNIQUES

Arch Segment Movements

The ability to move a group of teeth does not necessarily change the types of appliances that can be employed. Arch bars, lever arms, and the expansion screws can all be used to effect the movement of more than a single tooth. Arch bars are limited to the incisal areas for the most part, particularly the mandibular incisors. The usual situation is to combine the arch bar for effecting pressure on the segment and an acrylic plate to act as an anchorage device. Lever arms can be lengthened or positioned to affect a group of teeth at the same time. When applied in this manner, the lever arms are more effective if the points of expansion or compression along the active arm are multiple—that is, the arm makes two or more activating bends or utilizes more than one spring coil in the active component. The most common appliance used to move a segment of the dentition is the expansion unit. These can be positioned in an acrylic plate and the plate sectioned to effect almost any directional movement desired for any number of teeth desired. The expansion unit is most often applied to the maxillary incisors and/or canines.

Surgical Movements

There are situations in which prolonged orthodontic therapy can be avoided by the use of surgical procedures to effect tooth movement. There are two forms of surgical movement—a block, or segmental osseous resection, and a surgical creation of an alveolar socket. The surgical movement of the alveolar socket is actually a surgical tipping of a tooth. It must be accomplished before the apex of the root structure closes. The situation in which it can be utilized most effectively is when the maxillary canine tooth is displaced rostrally or even lies horizontally in the maxilla. The procedure consists of incising the soft tissue from the incorrect position along the planned transition path to the desired location. The dental elevator is then used to free the periodontal ligament from the alveolar crest toward the apex of the root. At least half the root length is freed. It may be necessary to remove some of the bone along the crest of the dental arch to the point of desired position. The tooth is very gradually forced to rotate into the new position. This rotation must be accomplished without moving the apex or, in other words, the tooth is rotated with the apex used as a pivot point. If the apical blood supply is disturbed during this movement, loss of the tooth is probable. The normal maximum age for accomplishing this surgical procedure is about 7 months of age. When the tooth is in its new position, it must be held there for a period of at least 2 weeks. This stabilization may be achieved by resuturing the soft tissue to hold the canine, using a light wire to ligate the canine to the opposite canine or to the second premolar, or using an acrylic plate to absolutely immobilize the canine. In some cases, the total distance may be impossible to achieve without risking disruption of the apical blood supply. The tooth may be moved as far as dared surgically, then the balance of the movement can be accomplished orthodontically. The use of orthodontic elastic ligature thread attached to the acrylic plate is most effective.

The movement of teeth, arch segments, or entire arches by surgical intervention takes several forms. The basis of these techniques is the cutting of the bone around or between the teeth roots so that healing involves osseous repair rather than periodontal structures. These techniques still carry a significant risk factor for the teeth. The procedure involves loss of major portions of blood supply to the block being moved. The easiest of these procedures is the changing of the length of the mandible via a bilateral resection of the mandible. This is usually a technique to shorten the mandible and is accomplished by removing the lower second premolar on each side. The mandible is then resected, on a buccal to lingual and rostral to caudal angle, around the mandibular canal, and the segments are overlapped to reduce mandibular length. The opposite can be done to lengthen the mandible. These procedures must be carefully planned on oral casts of the entire upper and lower arches.

Extreme care must be exercised in planning a block resection to move one or more teeth, usually in the incisal area. These roots lie very close to each other, the root structures converge toward the apex, and the contour of the anterior mandible and maxilla makes these techniques difficult to execute. After a block resection and movement, precise stabilization must be implemented for at least 4 to 6 weeks. The retaining splints also jeopardize tissue health by increasing the likelihood of periodontal disease during the time of osseous repair.

DESCRIPTIONS OF COMMON APPLIANCE TYPES

REMOVABLE MAXILLARY ACRYLIC PLATE

The acrylic plate forms the basis of a multitude of orthodontic appliances. The acrylic plate is best designed on an oral cast. The advantages of using a cast, rather than pouring the acrylic in the mouth, include greatly improved design ability, increased accuracy of pressure application, development of the appliance at a convenient time, ability to trim and polish the unit, ease of alterations, and avoidance of soft-tissue injury from the exothermic setting reaction of acrylic. The long-term comfort for the animal and reduction of soft-tissue irritation are made possible when the acrylic plate is used as a removable unit.

Almost all maxillary acrylic plates can be used as removable units. The easiest way to make the plate removable is to incorporate into the acrylic a small wire peg or hoop on the lingual surface of the teeth to be used to stabilize the plate. This is usually the maxillary canines and lateral incisors. The wire hoop is contoured to closely lie against the lingual tooth surface and to reach half to two thirds the length of the tooth. The free ends of the wire are turned back out into the area to be occupied by the acrylic. These ends should have several bends in the wire to increase the retention in the acrylic. The attachment to the tooth is achieved by placing a bracket on the buccal surface of each tooth. A small elastic is stretched over the tooth, over the wire hoop or peg, and over the top of the bracket. The size of the wire used to make the hoop will vary with the size of the dog, but a .022 to a .026 wire is usually preferred. Elastic size is most often one-eighth inch, 2 to 3 ounce. The other teeth can be used if needed or for unusual appliance design. The support teeth can be in either the support section of the plate (more likely) or in the active section (if really needed for stabilization).

Once the plate form is designed, force is applied to the unit:

1. The simplest type is the acrylic bite plane. A build-up of acrylic at the point of contact of a lower tooth or teeth allows the force of mastication to move the lower tooth along an incline plane cut into the acrylic. This type of appliance is particularly effective when used against the lower canines; it is of little value for the incisors.

2. The microscrew device can be embedded in the maxillary acrylic plate to force movement of a single tooth. The microscrew is a spring-loaded piston incorporated in the end of a threaded rod. The rod is screwed into a brass cuff embedded in the acrylic to hold the unit in position. The rod is turned, by a small screwdriver, 90 degrees every second or third day to move it through the brass cuff and increase the pressure on the spring-loaded piston. The spring in the piston reduces the discomfort that would occur if all the pressure created by turning the rod 90 degrees were transmitted to the tooth at one time. The spring absorbs the initial pressure and expands to keep the force on the tooth constant as the tooth moves.

This type appliance is most often used against the lingual surface of the incisors. It is possible to use more than one microscrew in a plate.

3. The expansion screw is similar in theory to the microscrew in that it allows the gradual movement of the force-exerting unit and diminishes changes in pressure on the affected teeth. Because the expansion screw utilizes an area of the acrylic plate to bring about force application, it can be used to move a group of teeth or an entire arch segment. In the appliance design, it is determined which teeth are to be moved and the expansion screw is positioned in the proper direction. After the acrylic hardens, a diamond disk is used to cut the segment that will move free from the rest of the plate. With half the expansion screw in the base and half in the active segment, the plate is ready to use.

4. Various types of anchorage units can be placed in the acrylic plate. The use of a loop or hook, from which an elastic can be stretched to a tooth or arch bar, makes it possible to spread the force of movement against the rest of the anterior maxilla. The use of larger wire allows the hook to be placed some distance from the acrylic and still use the plate as the anchorage. Similarly, springs and lever arms can be used against one or more teeth while the plate spreads the anchorage to both hard and soft tissue of the area. A tooth can act as both a point of retention of the plate and as a point of force or movement.

5. The acrylic unit can be used as a point of ligation, either with wire or elastic ligature thread. Small holes drilled in the plate at desired points allow either wire or thread to be used on individual teeth. Once the ligation is placed, it is usually good to cover these holes with added amounts of acrylic. The use of ligation techniques usually makes the plate into a nonremovable appliance.

MANDIBULAR ACRYLIC UNIT

Due to the difficulty in making the mandibular acrylic plate a removable unit, the technique has limited application in this area. The most frequent application is for extensive movement of the lower incisors. The acrylic plate serves as a base for hooks or spring levers in this area. The usual technique involves retraction of incisors using a lower segmental arch bar to equalize movement and maintain arch form. The acrylic plate is formed to cover the floor of the mouth from the rostral edge of the canines back to the second or third premolar on each side. The plate covers the premolar surfaces to let the teeth bear the pressure of a circum-mandibular wire between PM 1 and PM 2 on each side. Two hooks are positioned in the plate between the canines to attach elastics. A slight acrylic build-up behind the hooks prevents the ventral surface of the tongue from catching on these hooks.

RETAINERS

CONCEPT OF RETAINERS

The basic purpose of a retainer is to allow the oral structures to gain stability following movement via orthodontics or surgical procedures. If this period of adjustment is not provided for in the treatment planning, the probability of failure is very high. The amount of detail necessary to incorporate in the retainer phase of therapy varies with the amount and type of movements that have been done. The greater the interlocking action of the teeth in their new positions, the shorter the period of retainer utilization. Most orthodontic procedures require at least 4 to 6 weeks of retainer utilization to give a reasonable repair of the tissues affected by the orthodontic movement.

Quite frequently, a modification of the active unit can be created and the same basic appliance utilized as a retaining device. For instance, when an elastic ligature is used, it can be replaced with a light wire; the existing brackets may be utilized during the retainer time. When an acrylic appliance is used for movement, the portion applying a force can be neutralized or made passive, and the same acrylic unit made to function as a retainer. Occasionally, the movement of teeth is so extensive that new oral casts are needed to fabricate an appropriate retaining unit. Do not jeopardize the success of therapy by trying to cut short the retainer phase of therapy!

TIME REQUIREMENTS

From a technical point of view, the time required to accomplish orthodontic treatment is the same in the dog as it is in man, for the biomechanics of tooth movement are the same. From a practical point of view and from the standpoint of soft-tissue health, the time involved must be reduced to a minimum. Oral hygiene is critical during the time an appliance is in the mouth. Appliance design must minimize oral discomfort and soft-tissue irritation during therapy. If orthodontic treatment results in soft-tissue damage either through prolonged contact or improper design, the end result will be periodontal disease and early loss of teeth.

Most procedures should be completed in a few months. Most

cases require 1 to 3 months to accomplish the active stage of therapy and another month or two in retainers. The occasional case that requires a longer treatment period should be handled with great care, and every possible consideration should be given to soft-tissue protection. Removable appliances offer the best opportunity of minimizing orthodontic damage. The removal of the appliance for a few hours each day allows soft tissues to recover and repair most tissue insults.

TYPES OF DAMAGE

The most frequent types of damage seen during orthodontic therapy fall into four basic areas. Any foreign object (orthodontic bracket, band, or excess cement) positioned at or below the gingival margin will irritate the gingival tissue either by direct contact or by enhancing the accumulation of food debris, hair, and bacterial populations in immediate contact with the gingiva. The second area of damage in therapy is when orthodontic arch wire, elastics, springs, screws, and so forth contact the soft tissue and inflict pressure damage on the tissues. The third type of damage is when orthodontic appliances cover various amounts of oral soft tissue. These appliances, which are usually acrylic, tend to restrict the natural oral hygiene and accumulate debris. When the design of these units is less than correct and the unit applies pressure on the soft tissue, the irritation and restriction of blood flow result in tissue damage. This type of damage is compounded when the acrylic units are left in the mouth for extended periods without removal or cleaning, which does not allow the soft tissue time to rest and repair. The fourth type of damage is the application of improper force to the teeth themselves. Excessive pressure can move the tooth too fast and result in significant loosening of the tooth or movement of the tooth in an incorrect direction. Tooth position can be changed by treatment, but if the new position is achieved too fast or it compromises the function of that tooth, the end result is tooth or periodontal destruction.

ORTHODONTIC THERAPY PROBLEMS

A large percentage of treatment problems can be avoided by spending more time in the planning stages of therapy. Such evaluation factors as accurate application of force, path of tooth movement, and space requirements in the final position must be known to within a fraction of a millimeter if treatment is to progress smoothly.

When tooth movement occurs incorrectly in any dimension, when unnecessary occlusal trauma occurs during or after treatment, or when soft-tissue destruction accompanies treatment, the answer can usually be found by reviewing the original casts and appliances. The skill needed to make decisions based on fractions of a millimeter comes with practice; the patience to plan all stages of treatment comes from self discipline.

FREQUENTLY ENCOUNTERED PROBLEMS

Other than errors in appliance design and implementation, the most frequently encountered problem is loss of brackets. The precise adherence to instructions in placing direct bond brackets cannot be overemphasized or repeated too frequently. There *must* be a clean enamel surface; the enamel *must* be completely etched; the bracket base *must* be closely contoured to the tooth surface; the base and enamel *must* be free of all moisture and oil when the cement is applied; correct proportions of cement materials *must* be used; and the *exact* observations of time requirements in mixing, placement, and setting of the cement are essential. Direct bond brackets can be used effectively in the dog.

Certain factors involved in bracket loss, such as allergies, fuzzy chew items, excessive play with other animals, and chewing produced by boredom, can be controlled by the client. The continual chewing or licking of the skin seen with allergy problems results in catching the bracket in the hair and popping it off. The control of fleas, allergies, and other skin-irritating factors greatly reduces the likelihood of bracket loss. Removal of fuzzy items (rugs, toys, bedding) from the dog's environment obviously reduces the possibility of catching brackets in these items. Dry dog food may be a factor, but because few brackets are used on the posterior teeth, it is not of major concern.

Occasionally, individual teeth will be encountered that almost seem to refuse to hold a bracket. When repeat attempts fail to achieve a stable bond, an alternative is the use of "super" glue. Don't remove the remnants of the direct bond cement; just apply a single drop on the old bracket and reposition the bracket on the tooth. This technique can also be used by the client at home as a temporary repair until the bracket can be properly replaced. The "super" glue can be used repeatedly without damage to the tooth enamel.

Initial adaptation of the animal to the appliance may cause some concern for the owner and the animal. There are two approaches to this phase of therapy. Sedating the animal and allowing it to "wake-up" with the appliance in place works well for most animals. However, if resistance is encountered, it will last until the animal is completely out of the effects of sedation, and any attempts at correction of the inappropriate behavior will not be remembered after recovery. When appliances are difficult to position or have to be attached by ligature wires, this may be the only way. When a removable appliance is used, it is usually better to make the oral casts and place the brackets, allow the animal to recover from the anesthesia, and place the appliance for the first time with the animal fully awake. With this technique, the operator must be ready for a short period of intense resistance from the pet. A good choke chain and stout leash allow correction of any inappropriate behavior. Usually 15 to 30 minutes of adaptation time is all that is needed. Be sure to let the animal move at will, even though the leash is still attached during the last 10 to 15 minutes. If marked resistance is initially encountered, remove the appliance after it has been worn for 15 minutes without resistance and put it back in after 1 hour. Repeat this cycle until no objection is encountered.

Initial resistance to appliances usually takes the form to trying to remove the unit with the front paws. The paws must not be allowed in the mouth. Slight jerks on the leash may be all that are required, but the operator should be familiar with correct use of the choke chain in case more severe resistant is needed to stop the removal attempts. A few animals may require a muzzle or Elizabethan collar for 24 to 48 hours to accept the appliance. Sometimes the use of a wire ligature instead of the small elastic band for retention for the first 2 days gives enough appliance stability to convince the animal it cannot remove the unit. Under no circumstances should the animal learn that it can remove the appliance repeatedly by using its paws to rake the unit out of the mouth!

THERAPY-INDUCED PROBLEMS

Oral damage during therapy is the result of therapy design, material failure, lack of client observation, or patient-induced problems. The majority of problems can be traced to therapy design or its implementation! When appliances are designed and fit properly, negative patient response is rare. Failure of the client to closely monitor orthodontic therapy may allow a small problem to become severe.

The oral soft tissue suffers most frequently from orthodontic appliances. Elastics or wires that are allowed to put pressure on the gingiva will cut into the tissue in a short period of time. Acrylic units that aren't removed and cleaned regularly build accumulations of food and bacteria under the plate. Erosion of the oral epithelium under the plate is rapid. Permanent loss of epithelial pigmentation is the visual evidence of this type of tissue damage. Mobility of the acrylic unit and hair entrapment in the gingival crevice result in soft-tissue irritation.

Movement of teeth faster than the body can remodel the alveolar bone, and periodontal ligament will detach the ligament fibers and result in loosening of the teeth. Some loosening occurs with most movement of teeth; however, excessive tearing of these fibers can lead to periodontal disease or the immediate extraction of the tooth.

Occlusal trauma may result in structural loss, periodontal disease, and loss of alveolar bone when teeth are moved into incorrect positions. With incorrectly applied brackets or bands, there will occasionally be enamel damage. This most often takes the form of oral stains penetrating damaged enamel surfaces. The slip of an instrument or bur can destroy enamel as well as fracture teeth.

The animal's mouth usually does not completely repair itself when this damage occurs. Even though the tissue visually returns to normal, the damage at the structural level persists. The end result is an increased rate of periodontal problems and early loss of teeth. The vast majority of therapy-induced problems revolve around soft-tissue destruction. The use of permanently positioned acrylic appliances almost guarantees soft-tissue damage.

LONG-TERM EFFECTS OF THERAPY

The long-term effects of therapy are usually a balance between the benefits of improved occlusion and the periodontal damage suffered during therapy. The goal of orthodontic therapy is to maximize the benefits of having proper occlusion and to minimize the side effects. The whole concept of long-term benefits and limiting damage revolves around treatment planning and oral hygiene. Hygiene is essential during therapy and continues to be a significant factor in reducing periodontal disease throughout the animal's life.

Veterinary Dental Clinic
9695 S.W. Freeway
Houston, Texas 77074

Dentistry   0195–5616/86 $0.00 + .20

Orthodontics for the Dog

Bite Evaluation, Basic Concepts, and Equipment

*Donald L. Ross, D.V.M., M.S.**

The reasons for small animal orthodontic therapy are almost identical to those for orthodontic therapy in man. The problems introduced by abnormal occlusion include those of only minimal esthetic importance to those that can limit life expectancy. Fortunately, nature can adapt almost any erupting dental pattern to a form that will at least sustain life. The problem then becomes one of identifying abnormalities and categorizing the anomalies in groups relative to their physiologic, genetic, and esthetic importance. Then the veterinarian can offer logical choices to the client based on a knowledge of the problems present, their origin, and their likely long-term effects on each animal.

As occlusal abnormalities are followed over succeeding generations, it becomes apparent that correct diagnosis is essential to the oral health of the individual and, through selection, the correct oral function of future generations. From the standpoint of the individual animal, the most frequently seen problems result in periodontal disease and subsequent tooth loss. As occlusal problems increase in severity, the ability to ingest certain forms of foodstuffs becomes impaired. More severe problems can reduce not only types of food eaten but also the volume that can be ingested. The systemic effects of bacterial invasion, secondary to occlusal abnormalities, become almost a study within themselves, whether the invasion comes via induced periodontal disease or via the pulp chamber after fracture of the crown structure.

The dentition affects the appearance of the entire facial area. Because the dog can open its mouth widely, there are many more teeth visible. The aesthetic aspects of minor abnormalities are often

---

*Veterinary Dental Clinic, Houston, Texas

of greater significance to the client than the affect of these abnormalities on the animal's health. For the client involved in conformation or obedience competition, minor problems often assume massive proportions. Even the pet owner that closely interacts with an animal will often detect occlusal problems and inquire about their significance or correction.

ORAL EVALUATION

The occlusion of the carnivore is basically the same, whether the animal is a domestic cat or a large bear. The effective use of the muscles of mastication and bone structure of the facial region has not been improved over the years by man's selective breeding. The deviations toward the prognathic or brachygnathic breeds have always led to increased oral problems via traumatic occlusal patterns, increased occurrence of peridontal problems, and altered respiratory function. Hence, a precise understanding of the correct canine occlusion is necessary for a precise evaluation of the dentition.

Unfortunately, breed standards go no farther in the description of the correct canine occlusion than to state the relationship of the incisors and the number of teeth that should be present. The incisors do not give a complete picture of the occlusion of an individual and should be only the first step in bite evaluation. Although it is obvious that the maxillary incisors should overlap the mandibular incisors, the degree of overlap and position of each incisor should be noted. The large cusp or tubercle of the mandibular central incisors should contact the lingual surface of the maxillary incisors at the base or cingulum. This relationship is approximately centered so that one tooth is directly in front of the other. The mandibular intermediates and laterals gradually lose the centered-type relationship. At the lower laterals, the large cusp should be in the interproximal space in front of its maxillary counterpart.

The incisor's root structure is relatively small when compared with many other teeth, and the bone structure on the facial surface is thin. Being on the leading edge of the facial structures, the incisors frequently absorb direct traumatic insults. This combination of lack of root size and bone support and increased environmental pressures often results in positional changes of the incisors that are mistakenly taken for structural abnormalities. The fact that the upper and lower jaws do not always develop in perfect synchronization may lead to occlusal problems. When the teeth erupt (either deciduous or permanent) in an incorrect occlusal position because of spurts of jaw growth in either jaw, they tend to maintain the occlusal position under the influence of the forces of mastication. All factors considered, to look at the incisors alone is very misleading when attempting genetic evaluation by phenotype.

More reliable guides or additional reference points would include the canines, premolars (both rostral/caudal and horizontal relationships), and the relationship between the temperomandibular joint (TMJ) and the angle of the mandible. The mandibular canine represents one of the most stable reference points in the mouth. Because limited positional changes are possible in cases of minor genetic abnormalities, more importance should be given to minor shifts in the lower canine and its relation to the maxillary canine lateral incisor. Ideally, the lower canine should fit exactly between the maxillary canine and lateral incisor, with equal space between the lower canine and each upper tooth. The rostral/caudal relationship of the premolars is such that the large cusp of the mandibular premolar points exactly into the interproximal space in *front* of its maxillary counterpart. In the horizontal plane, the cusp tips of the premolars should overlap at least as far forward as the tips of the second premolars. The angle of the mandible is ideally positioned directly below the posterior edge of the articulating surface of the mandibular condyle.

Three other areas should be noted during an occlusal evaluation of the animal. The first is that all points considered to be midline of the head (occipital crest, midpoint between the eyes, midpoint of the nose pad, and the midpoint of both dental arches) lie along the same vertical plane. The next is the relationship of the width of the mandible to the maxilla. The lower jaw must be wide enough at the canine teeth to allow these teeth to flair laterally slightly and close without putting pressure on the maxillary soft tissue. The last, while having little to do with the actual occlusion, is important in terms of the longevity of the lower central incisors. The floor of the mouth, between the canine teeth, should be relatively flat. The presence of a groove or depression along the midline indicates the presence of excess cartilage between the mandibles. When the lower central incisors have insufficient bone support to maintain correct occlusal position, the teeth drop down and tilt forward as the animal ages.

OCCLUSAL EVALUATION TABLE

The development of a chart of oral evaluation has often been suggested as a means of uniformly rating the genetics of the mouth. The chart (Table 1) has been tried in the breeding programs of several large breeds and is presented here to encourage constructive criticism and evaluation. Score each area and add the scores for a final point total.

Table 1. Oral Evaluation Chart

I. Incisor Relationship (Value of 5 Points)
   A. If lower incisors hit the cingulum of the uppers (a "scissor" bite).   5
   B. If lower incisors are hitting the cusp tips of the uppers or hitting gingival
      tissue behind the uppers.   4
   C. If lowers are in front of uppers or are behind the uppers with space
      between upper and lower incisors.   3
   D. Marked space between upper and lower incisors.   2
   E. Extreme difference in jaw lengths.   1

II. Canine Tooth Relationship (Value of 5 Points)
   A. Lower canines centered between and not touching either upper canine or
      lateral incisor.   5
   B. Touching either upper tooth.   4
   C. Wearing of either upper tooth or downward angulation of incisor group so
      that lower canine tip touches upper canine and its base hits upper lateral
      incisor.   3
   D. Either inside or outside of upper canine or lateral incisor.   2
   E. Behind upper canine or ahead of upper lateral incisor.   1

III. Lower Fourth Premolar (Value of 5 Points)
   A. The large cusp tip is centered between the upper third and fourth
      premolar.   5
   B. Lower cusp tip shifts to the small third groove in upper third premolar or
      back to the front edge of upper fourth premolar.   4
   C. Lower cusp tip shifts to the middle groove in upper third premolar or
      back onto surface of upper fourth premolar.   3
   D. Lower cusp tip shifts to large first groove in upper third premolar or half
      the distance to cusp tip of upper fourth premolar.   2
   E. Lower cusp tip shifts to meet the cusp tip of either upper third or fourth
      premolar.   1

IV. Premolar Horizontal Alignment (Value of 5 Points)
   A. Interdigitation of cusp tips as far forward as the lower second premolar
      with upper second.   5
   B. Lower third premolar with the upper third.   4
   C. Lower fourth premolar with upper third.   3
   D. Space between tips of lower fourth and upper third.   2

V. TMJ Angle of Mandible Relationship (Value of 5 Points)
   A. Angle directly below posterior border of coronoid process or within 3 mm
      of that point.   5
   B. Angle displaced by 4 to 6 mm from point below posterior border of
      coronoid process.   4
   C. Angle displaced by 7 to 10 mm from point below posterior border of the
      coronoid process.   3
   D. More than 10-mm displacement from point below posterior border of the
      coronoid process.   2

VI. Head Symmetry (Value of 5 Points)
   A. Perfect midline of head and dentition alignment.   5
   B. Subtract one point for:
      1. Rotated teeth (either premolars or incisors).
      2. Midline of upper and lower arches off center by less than width of
         upper incisor.   4
      3. Missing one tooth.
   C. Subtract two points for:
      1. Rotated teeth in premolar and incisor areas.
      2. Midline off by width of one tooth.
      3. Missing two teeth.   3
   D. Subtract three points for:
      1. Midline off by more than width of one tooth.
      2. More than two missing teeth.
      3. Noticeable deviation of muzzle to left or right of midline of rest of
         skull.   2

Table 1. *Oral Evaluation Chart* Continued

Area Scores and Reasons (30 Points Possible):

A. Incisors	( )	_____
B. Canines	( )	_____
C. Fourth Premolar	( )	_____
D. Horizontal Alignment	( )	_____
E. Angle of Mandible	( )	_____
F. Oral Symmetry	( )	_____

Total Points =

Grade Scale:

Excellent (27–30 points): No apparent genetic defects.

Near Normal (21–26 points): Mild genetic problems; select mates with equal or better oral evaluation scores.

Genetic Defect (16–20 points): Careful use if other body traits warrant use in breeding program.

Severe Defect (0–15 points): Not suitable for breeding purposes.

GROWTH PATTERNS OF THE HEAD

In understanding growth patterns and explaining them to clients, it is helpful to use the following analogy even though it is not entirely ideologically correct. Consider the bone to be somewhat elastic in response to the interlock of the upper and lower teeth and the forces exerted by elongation growth. If mandibular growth is considered to come from the condylar region and elongation forces the mandibular development down and forward, it is easier to correlate the changes in mandibular form with the genetic abnormalities that produce growth deviations. Thus, when extra jaw length is inherited, the first change noted is the forward shift of the premolars, canines, and incisors to the extent the interlocking action of the two arches will allow. Beyond that, the following changes begin to occur. The body of the mandible begins to curve ventrally, and there is visible increase in space between the cusp tips of the premolars. The angle of the mandible begins a posterior shift in response to the limitation of forward movement by the lower canine against the maxillary lateral incisor. The lower incisors shift forward to come to an end-to-end relationship, which is called a "level bite" by breeders and show enthusiasts. A strong growth push is required to entirely overcome the occlusal interlock. When the mandibular canines move either lingual or buccal to the maxillary lateral incisors, the genetic defect is very serious. The complete extent of the genetic problem is determined by the addition of the degree of anterior displacement, the degree of mandibular curvature, and the amount of distal shift present in the angle of the mandible. To evaluate only a single area (the incisors) leads to erroneous characterizations of the genetic potential of individuals.

When discussing the opposite growth pattern, brachygnathism, the same general principles apply. The lack of mandibular growth, compared with the growth of the maxilla, results in the increase in space between the upper and lower incisors, the maxillary canine moves ahead to contact the caudal edge of the mandibular canine, the upper premolars drift over the top of their mandibular counterparts, and the angle of the mandible moves forward of the condyle. Thus, when the mandibular canines change their position in relation to the upper canine, a severe genetic abnormality is overriding the mechanics of the normal occlusion. It is the shift of the angle of the jaw that allows a severely affected animal to maintain a reasonable dental relationship at the expense of the effectiveness of the muscles of mastication. It is the canine-to-canine interlock and the mandibular first molar ahead of the maxillary first molar that mechanically force this shift in the angle-to-condyle relationship.

It is important to note that effect of the mechanical interlocking action of teeth can act to maintain an incorrect occlusal pattern when no genetic abnormality exists as easily as it can act to prevent the loss of normal occlusion in the presence of a genetic defect. The most notable example of this occurs when the deciduous teeth erupt in an incorrect pattern in the young puppy. This usually occurs as a result of a lack of synchronization of upper and lower jaw development prior to eruption of the deciduous dentition. When the deciduous teeth are removed in the 6- to 10-week-old individuals having canines or incisors in an improper position, the jaw structure will correct if there is no genetic abnormality.

CONCEPTS OF ORTHODONTICS

HOW TEETH MOVE

The biomechanical basis of orthodontic procedures is that teeth can be moved through bone if the supporting tissues (primarily the alveolar bone and periodontal ligament) are given time to reorganize during the movement process. Changes in tension on the periodontal ligament fibers are created when pressure on the crown of the tooth is transmitted down the root to the ligament fibers. The body responds to changes in ligament fiber tension by trying to equalize the tension around the diameter of the root. In areas of decreased ligament tension, the body resorbs alveolar bone. In areas of increased tension, the body deposits new alveolar bone. When the pressure on the ligament fibers exceeds the ability of the body to change bone configuration, the ligament fibers begin to separate from the bone, and if the process continues, the teeth become loose in the alveolar socket. Extraction of teeth is possible from excessive orthodontic pressure.

The fact that pressure applied to the teeth creates forces in all three dimensions must be kept in mind when designing appliances. Close analysis of all force vectors cannot be overemphasized. The tip of the tooth root may act as a pivot point or the alveolar bone crest may act as a fulcrum. Without the benefit of models in which techniques can be tested on artificial teeth embedded in wax, experience becomes important. Start with simple problems, observe cases closely and regularly, and study the various techniques available for handling similar problems.

LENGTH OF TREATMENT

In human orthodontics, it is not unusual for it to take 2 to 3 years to complete tooth movements. There are several reasons why this is not practical in the dog. In most cases, therapy should be completed in 3 to 6 months. The majority of canine problems that are responsive to orthodontic threatment involve the incisors and/or the canines, and when therapy is limited to these areas, it can be effected in a reasonable amount of time. Among other reasons for completing therapy as soon as possible is the fact that the levels of oral hygiene usually are not as high in the dog as in man. The lack of oral hygiene results in oral soft-tissue irritation, periodontal disease, and, frequently, unrepairable soft-tissue damage. The use of materials designed for human usage almost guarantees some degree of irritation.

Limitation of treatment time, use of removable orthodontic units, and strong emphasis on oral hygiene give the best possibility of minimizing oral damage from therapy. It may be desirable to move teeth rapidly enough to result in some mobility at the end of movement in order to minimize the damage from appliances. The teeth can re-establish integrity of the periodontal ligaments during the retainer application. The balance of the various types of damage becomes difficult at times and emphasizes the extreme importance of closely monitoring therapy when active appliances are in the mouth.

LIMITS TO MOVEMENT

There are physical limits to the movement of teeth. The maxillary and mandibular osseous structure will allow movement of the teeth through any portion, but there are areas that will not support the teeth if movement goes that far. The obvious limits of the cortical plates of the mandible, the lateral plate of the maxilla, and the nasal passage of the maxilla need little justification as a limit to tooth movement. Once the tooth root penetrates, either with total body movement or with tippage of the root tip or crown, the stability of the tooth diminishes quickly. The less obvious limits are provided by such factors as the occlusal interaction with the opposite arch. This is most notable in the canine and carnassial teeth of either arch. Mandibular and maxillary incisors face a limit in any lingual movement produced by a reduction of arch length as the incisors collapse inward. When the total width of the teeth equals the space available, movement must stop or the teeth will begin to crowd and rotate. Extreme care must be used in planning orthodontic movement to ensure the space is available to accomplish the needed changes. Casts of the dentition are invaluable tools in treatment planning because they allow accurate measurements of these distances. The basic decision of tooth movement is the determination of available space in the desired location.

EQUIPMENT AND MATERIALS

The instrumentation and materials required in most orthodontic techniques are relatively small. Other than the initial investment in the hand instruments, the costs are also small. Start with the basics and add both equipment and materials as the individual cases require.

BASIC HAND INSTRUMENTS

The types of pliers available to manipulate wire are legion, and one's choice of a basic set depends much on individual preference. A suggestion would be to start with the following: tweed arch pliers, bird-beak pliers, three-stage loop-forming pliers, clasp-adjusting pliers, wire cutters (for ligature wire and for wire up to 0.036), and bracket-removing pliers.

Other necessary hand instruments include a ligature tucker, a pair of cotton forceps, mosquito forceps, large needle holders for twisting wire, and a wax carrier-carver. A Bunsen burner is needed for annealing wire and flowing wax.

Handpiece Accessories (The Handpiece Should Be Straight)

Burs are necessary in several stages of many orthodontic techniques. The bur sizes one is likely to need include the round sizes

#1/2, 1, 2, 4, 6, and 8; the tapered cones #699, 701, and 703; and the acrylic burs in round and flame shapes.

Disks are loosely described here as those accessories that are used with a mandrel (usually a #303 mandrel). They would include the safe-sided diamond disk (thin, semirigid, and 1/2-inch diameters), polishing disks (either brush or rag), sandpaper disks, and abrasive wheels.

For polishing, flour of pumice paste and rubber polishing cups are used to prepare enamel for direct bonding cements.

WIRES

Orthodontic wire is available in a multitude of types and sizes. For most applications, the dead-soft round wire is sufficient. The typical sizes needed for the dog would include .018, .022, .026, and .030 diameters. These usually come in 12-inch lengths, and there are 10 pieces per container. In theory, "round" wire is harder to use for precise tooth control than the "square" wire; however, its ease of manipulation makes it a good wire to utilize during the learning stages. To gain skill in the "art" of developing wire appliances, draw a 4- to 6-inch line on a piece of paper. Put several bends, curves, and loops in the line and then bend a wire length to match the line on the paper. It should match the line exactly and lie perfectly flat on the paper when done properly.

The term "dead-soft" refers to the lack of resiliency or "memory" in the wire. When bent, the wire stays bent and has no tendency to return to its original shape. For wire to be effective in orthodontic therapy, it must have some resilience to be able to apply pressure to teeth or be able to withstand pressure of teeth that don't move easily. This is done by heating the wire, after the desired shape has been obtained, until it is a very light tan color. *Great care must be used not to heat the wire until it is red hot or it will lose all resiliency forever.* The wire should be passed through the Bunsen burner flame rapidly for several passes until the light tan color is achieved. With experience, the wire can be left in the flame for longer periods of time to achieve the annealing effect.

ELASTICS

Elastics are used to apply pressure to teeth and hold appliances in proper position. They are supplied in a wide variety of sizes and strengths. The normal forces used in canine orthodontics range from 1 to 3 ounces. Elastic strength is measured by expanding the elastic to three times its resting diameter and measuring the pressure at that point. The most frequently used sizes are 1/8, 3/16, 1/4, 5/16, and 3/8 inches and these in strengths of 2 ounces and 3 or 3.5 ounces. Extreme care must be exercised when using elastics in orthodontic procedures. When elastics break, slip out of position, or are left on too long, the damage can be extensive and sometimes permanent. When contacting the oral tissue, they can cut the soft tissue or bone. When excessive force is applied to the teeth at an incorrect angle, or applied for extended periods, movement in the wrong direction, elevation, depression, rotation, or even extraction of the teeth can occur.

Two other elastic products that are useful in canine procedures are the elastic string and the elastic ligatures. The elastic string is available in light, medium, and heavy sizes. Applications include tooth ligation, appliance retention, and for pressure application in areas where correct size elastics are not available. The elastic ligature is a small elastic ring that slips over the orthodontic bracket to hold appliances in the bracket.

ACRYLICS

Orthodontic acrylic is a polymethyl methacrylate and may be used to form the basis of either an active appliance or a retainer. The product is supplied as a powder (the polymer) and a liquid (the monomer) that, when mixed and hardened, form the acrylic material. The acrylic appliances are almost always formed on an oral cast to avoid tissue damage from the exothermic reaction of acrylic curing, because of the ease of appliance design and accuracy of development. The versatility of acrylics is demonstrated by the ability to modify the unit in so many ways. If an area is thin, more powder and liquid can be added. If the acrylic is too thick, portions can be removed. Holes can be drilled for attachment, various pressure-producing units can be attached or imbedded, and the forms are limitless.

BRACKETS

The types of brackets necessary for most orthodontic applications are rather small. In fact, the straight slot bracket designed for the human mandibular central incisor, slotted for 0.22 wire, will probably accomplish almost any canine orthodontic procedure. The most common situation is to have this bracket attached to bracket bases of several sizes to accommodate the various breeds and tooth sizes. The mandibular central base is the smallest of the human bracket bases and can be used for most dogs. A larger base may be needed for use on the canine teeth. The versatility, ease of use, and tolerance by oral tissue make the direct bond technique the one of choice for almost all canine work.

CEMENTS

The use of the direct bonding cements vastly expands the orthodontic techniques for the dog. These cements must be used precisely or the maintenance problems will discourage their routine usage. The ability to quickly apply brackets to teeth will decrease the preparation time, increase the use of removable appliances, and make changing appliances during therapy easier. There are several brand names available, some with a chemical activator and some that are light-cured. The chemically activated bonding agents are recommended, for even though the working time is limited, the setting reaction occurs under the bracket where no light-cured cement can be activated. There are two basic rules that must be adhered to regardless of whether the cement is chemical- or light-activated: the first is that the area and all materials must be kept free of contamination by moisture or oils; the second is that the acid etch of the enamel must be thorough, and this usually means increasing the length of time the acid is left on the tooth surface by 1.5 to 2 times the recommended time for human teeth. These cements bond by chemical interaction with the enamel and mechanically sealing within the minute irregularities between the bracket and the tooth surface. Neither of these actions can occur if the bracket is not closely contoured to the surface of the tooth and if absolute cleanliness and dryness are not maintained during the bonding process.

The use of the older cement forms that bond only by mechanical retention requires the use of the orthodontic band. These bands require considerable skill to develop and cement properly. The bands are individually fabricated for each tooth from strips of band material, the bracket is welded to the band, and then the unit is cemented in place. In most cases, a dental lab is used to develop the bands and appliances. The potential for soft-tissue irritation or damage from the band and bracket combination and the excess cement that frequently is left during the cementation process is much greater than with the direct bonding procedures.

When properly applied, the orthodontic band has greater strength than the direct bonding bracket. However, this difference in strength is of little significance when the orthodontic forces are kept within acceptable limits and appliances are properly designed.

With both types, there will be times when the cement will fail and the unit will have to be replaced. It is quicker and easier to replace a direct bond unit with a new unit than it is to reshape and reuse the old band and bracket combination.

SOURCES OF SUPPLIES

The major suppliers of orthodontic materials include Rocky Mountain Orthodontics, Unitek, Lee Pharmaceuticals, J&J, and 3M. Most of these retail through local dental supply houses. A personal favorite for direct bonding cement is Reliance Orthodontic Cement from Reliable Dental Supply and the Lok-Mesh Bracket Bases from Rocky Mountain.

Veterinary Dental Clinic
9695 S. W. Freeway
Houston, Texas 77074

0195–5616/86 $0.00 + .20

Oral Surgery

Basic Techniques

Donald L. Ross, D.V.M., M.S.,*
and Gary S. Goldstein, D.V.M.†

The surgical techniques for the oral cavity can range from the relatively simple to the very complex in the attempts to improve health, function, and appearance. Quite often there is more than one way to solve similar problems. The ability of the individual to handle surgical situations depends on accurate evaluation of the case, knowledge of the options available, and refinement of surgical skills through practice. Some of the clinical problems seen most frequently and their surgical solutions will be discussed. Obviously, all techniques for all problems would become a textbook rather than an attempt to give the practitioner what is needed to meet 95 per cent of the clinical cases encountered.

EXTRACTION OF TEETH

The frequency of tooth extraction for the small animal patient is so great that it is important to have a very clear idea of the reasons for removal of either deciduous or permanent teeth. It is clearly recognized that client attitude plays more of a role in reasons for extraction of teeth than in most other aspects of oral care. When the biological principles of tooth health have been evaluated, then client evaluation will often affect the surgical recommendations. Deciduous teeth and permanent teeth are usually extracted for very different reasons.

*Veterinary Dental Clinic, Houston, Texas
†Veterinary Dental Clinic, Houston, Texas

Deciduous Teeth

Potential reasons for extraction of deciduous teeth begin almost as soon as the teeth erupt, or fail to erupt, into the oral cavity. In the 6- to 8-week-old animal, reasons for extraction would include malpositions, unequal jaw lengths, dental cysts, tooth fractures, and fractures of the maxilla or mandible. Failure to remove teeth in the young individual, where indicated, will create permanent occlusal, periodontal, or structural problems. In the 4- to 6-month-old animal, reasons for deciduous extractions usually involve a lack of root resorption of the deciduous tooth. Again, failure to promptly extract deciduous teeth when root resorption and exfoliation are delayed will lead to occlusal abnormalities and early onset of periodontal disease.

Extraction of deciduous teeth requires close attention to detail because of the anatomy of the deciduous tooth. In general, the root structure tends to be proportionally slimmer and longer in the deciduous tooth than in the permanent tooth. Along with the resorptive process that removes dentin from the root as the animal ages, the shape of the root lends itself to fractures at the base of the crown when extraction forceps are used as the primary instrument. This anatomy makes the elevator the primary instrument for removal of these teeth. The diameter of the working tip of the elevator should be between one quarter and one half the diameter of the root structure. Initially, the tip of the instrument is used to sever the fibers of the periodontal ligament down to the crest of the alveolar bone. Then the tip is gradually forced, a few millimeters at a time, into the alvelar socket around the circumference of the root. By rotating the instrument, periodontal ligament fibers are torn and alveolar bone is fractured. Care should be exercised in rotating the elevator in the alveolar socket, for the wall of the deciduous tooth root is often thin and will fracture under pressure. As the elevator is pushed deeper into the socket, the root becomes thinner. A few extra seconds spent with the elevator is much safer than applying rotational forces with extraction forceps. When working with the deciduous premolars, the teeth should be cut into individual root segments with a small round dental bur if both root structures are intact.

The age of the animal should be kept in mind when removing deciduous teeth. In the 6- to 12-week-old animals, the root of the deciduous tooth is in very close proximity to the developing crown of the permanent tooth. The epithelial tissue that deposits the enamel over the crown of the forming tooth is only one-cell thick. Elevators allowed to contact this tissue and the newly formed enamel result in permanent enamel defects when the tooth erupts. These areas usually appear as small pits in the enamel that tend to absorb oral debris (stain) easily. Composite restorative material can be used to fill these lesions, but prevention is certainly preferable. Much more time should be spent rotating the tooth with the elevator only partially inserted in the alveolar socket; try to avoid carrying the instrument any deeper than necessary.

One should remember that many fractured deciduous root tips do not resorb. They are maintained in the alveolar bone, continuing to displace the permanent tooth for extended periods of time before being abscessed out of the bone. Every reasonable effort should be made to remove these fractured root tips. Postponing deciduous extraction is rarely a correct decision. The quicker the offending tooth is removed, the easier it is for the permanent tooth to assume its normal position. Soft-tissue damage is to be avoided during extraction procedures. Bone will repair routinely, but the delicate tissue of the gingival crevice often sustains damage that does not completely repair in the healing process.

PERMANENT TEETH

Extraction of the permanent teeth differs from removal of deciduous teeth in that the root structure is a much stronger entity and can absorb more pressure without fracturing. Even the permanent tooth root is not as strong as the combined strength of the periodontal ligament fibers. Therefore, the goal of any technique is to stretch, break, or cut small numbers of fibers at a time until enough have been destroyed to allow the safe removal of the tooth. Most extraction techniques begin with the tip of the elevator being used to cut the periodontal ligament fibers down to the crest of the alveolar bone.

At this point, one method is to push the tip of the elevator down into the alveolar socket. As the elevator is gradually worked into the periodontal ligament space, it cuts the fibers around the circumference of the root and displaces the root out of the socket. Applying rotational pressures while the tip is in the socket and parallel to the long axis of the root is also used to break ligament fibers. When the root is moving freely in the socket, the appropriate extraction forcep is used to break the last small number of fibers and remove the tooth.

Another approach to elevator application is to position the instrument perpendicular to the long axis of the root at the level of the alveolar crest. Rotating the elevator forces one cutting edge into the tooth and elevates the tooth as the elevator rests on bone. Pressure is applied in gradual increments and repeated rapidly.

Using the elevator in this manner around the circumference of the tooth root applies an elevating or lifting pressure against the periodontal ligament fibers in line with the elevator. Initial efforts will appear to have little effect. As the process continues, the tooth will gradually loosen in its socket, small amounts of hemorrhage will become visible as the fibers tear, and, finally, the tooth will loosen to the point that the extraction forceps can be safely used to finsih the extraction process.

In almost all cases, it is worth the time and effort to section any multi-rooted tooth into its component parts and work against only one root at a time. Other techniques associated with the extraction process that either speed extraction or healing would include the reflection of the gingival tissue, reducing the height of the alveolar bone, and suturing of the gingival tissue to close the site (if marked infection is not present). The tissue glues offer a quick method of closing the soft tissue over an extraction site.

Removal of the canine teeth offers a challenge in extraction procedures. Often it is difficult to remove these teeth with the usual elevator techniques. Resection of the buccal alveolar bone is easily done with a dental bur and creates a simple extraction situation. The procedure begins by incising the soft tissue above the first premolar and parallel to the long axis of the canine. A soft-tissue flap is raised to completely expose the canine eminence. Using a dental bur, cut the buccal plate of bone along the rostral and caudal edge of the tooth and apically at least two thirds of the length of the root. Then extend the cut across the buccal surface of the tooth at the apical end of the other cuts. This not only removes the buccal plate of bone as a retentive factor but also produces a groove along the margin of the root. The elevator has an excellent purchase point along the groove to gradually break the remaining lingual ligament fibers. After removal of the tooth, the soft tissue can be repositioned and sutured to achieve first-intention healing.

SURGICAL REPOSITIONING OF TEETH

This terminology can be applied to two different procedures: the disruption of the alveolar socket and forcing relocation of a tooth or the sectioning of bone incorporating a tooth or group of teeth to move the block to a new position. The first technique is employed more often but must be done during the time of root formation and prior to closure of the root apex. The block resection technique is theoretically applicable in the mature animal, but the anatomy of the incisor/canine area makes it difficult to use.

In the 5- to 7-month-old animal, the displaced canine teeth are the most frequent candidates for surgical repositioning. The procedure consists of using the dental elevator to sever the periodontal ligament down to the crest of the alveolar bone. A scalpel blade cuts the soft tissue to the bone depth, from the caudal edge of the canine to the first premolar. The elevator is directed into the alveolar socket to approximately one third to one half the length of the root. This process loosens the tooth, fragments the alveolar bone, and allows the tooth to be gradually forced into the correct position. Care must be used to avoid severing the apical blood supply or completely detaching the tooth. Usually the shaft of the elevator can be gradually forced between the canine and lateral incisor. By rocking the elevator and slowly putting pressure on the canine, the tooth is moved caudally.

Stabilization is necessary to prevent the tooth from shifting back to the original position. Closing the soft tissue rostral to the repositioned tooth with mattress sutures may be adequate, but frequently it is necessary to wire the canine to the second premolar. This is done by putting the wire through the root bifurcation of the second premolar and back around the canine.

Occasionally, it is impossible to move the tooth all the way to the proper position with pressure. In these cases, move the tooth as far as possible and substitute orthodontic elastic ligature thread for the wire. The remaining movement is accomplished orthodontically over a period of a few weeks. Better to be a little conservative than to extract the tooth with too much force.

About 10 per cent of these cases will be less than totally successful. The problems will range from inability to achieve correct position to tooth discoloration from loss of blood supply to extraction of the tooth. Be very sure the apex has not closed when the procedure is attempted. Clients must be made aware that most of these cases can be handled with orthodontic techniques without as much risk if they are willing to wait until the animal's teeth are fully erupted.

TOOTH TRANSPLANT

To move teeth from a donor to a recipient may offer the simplest method of restoring oral function and appearance in some circumstances. As with organ transplants, this procedure is subject to failure, and when a tooth transplant is not successful, it can't be repeated. The obvious benefits in terms of function, maintenance, and appearance of natural tooth units make the technique highly desirable, but failure rates of at least 20 to 40 per cent are normal. Client awareness of all options is imperative prior to attempting this procedure.

Most often transplants are suggested when the natural tooth is broken at or below the gingival margin or fracture lines exit into the root area. In these cases, just a few options exist—extraction, transplant, or osseous implant. The most successful of the osseous implant techniques requires a year or more to complete and very intensive oral hygiene to maintain. Extraction leaves a vacancy in the dental arch. The transplant offers quick success (or failure) and the potential for complete restoration of appearance.

Successful transplants depend on avoiding host rejection. The procedures differ among authors. The minimum preparation of the transplant tooth consists of complete debridement of the tooth root, removing all periodontal ligament fibers and cementum. Most techniques also suggest that one open the tooth at the apex of the root and perform a root canal filling prior to implantation. Endodontically treated, frozen teeth have also been utilized successfully, which raises the possibility of a frozen "tooth bank."

Personal experience indicates that structural compatibility of the transplant tooth with the host alveolar socket, extraction techniques for both the transplant and the remaining host root, and postoperative stability are of paramount importance. If the tooth is removed from the donor without damage or nicks in the dentin, if no minute fractures are created in the host alveolar socket, if the root exactly fits the new socket or is a fraction of a millimeter larger, and if absolute stability is provided during the healing period, the success rates are very good. Debridement of the tooth root seems to be adequate preparation, but one cannot argue with the biological principles of endodontically treating the tooth to reduce the amount of foreign protein being introduced in the host system.

Methods of transplant stabilization may vary from simple suturing of the soft tissue to interdental wiring to bonding to adjacent teeth with composite restorative materials to an intraoral acrylic splint. The tooth must be held immobile for at least 2 weeks and longer if the stabilizing materials are not irritating oral soft tissue. During the healing period, absolute cleanliness is necessary and antibiotic coverage should be considered.

In selecting a donor animal, the biological process of tooth development should be kept in mind. The young animal will have a large pulp area and a relatively small amount of dentin to support future oral stress. The tooth of the older animal will have a greater percentage of dentin for tooth strength, but the reduced amounts of pulpal tissue may reduce the body fluid circulating in the tooth; drying will increase the likelihood of tooth fracture. Ideally, the tooth donor should be about 3 or 4 years of age, regardless of the age of the host.

ORAL ABSCESSES OF TOOTH ORIGIN

Abscesses that develop because of the presence of abnormal tooth structure are usually one of three types. The periodontal disease process that begins as a peridontal pocket, proceeds to alveolar osteitis, and ends as a purulent evulsion of the tooth constitutes the majority of these problems. Fractures of the tooth crown, pulpal hemorrhage, and root fractures (where the tooth remains in place) that lead to the bacterial invasion of the pulp chamber and periapical abscessation are the second type. The third type is the foreign-body response originating from root fragments in the alveolar bone. This can be produced by traumatic loss of the crown and portions of the root or by incomplete extraction of the root structure.

The typical response of the body to the presence of a root fragment is similar to that produced by a foreign body embedded in tissue. If the fragment is small, resorption is possible. The more frequent sequence of events is the establishment of a small chronic abscess around the fragment. If left undisturbed, the abscess will create a draining fistula into the oral cavity. After a period of several months, the fragment will eventually be evulsed from the dental arch. During the abscess period, the opening of the fistula will appear as a small, raised, reddened area on the gingiva or mucosa. A few root fragment abscesses in the lower jaw will drain ventrally through the skin.

Most root fragments can be easily located and removed. A gingival incision over the site occupied by the original tooth, reflection of the gingiva away from the old alveolar sockets, and elevation of the offending root fragment are usually easier than extraction of an intact tooth. By the time the drainage develops, much of the original periodontal ligament attachment has been destroyed, and the fragment is pushed from the bone by the abscess process. Occasionally, root fragments will have been displaced by the original trauma or extraction efforts. Radiographs can be used to pinpoint the location of the fragment and facilitate its removal.

IMPACTION OF TEETH

The surgical techniques appropriate for impacted teeth vary with the stage of tooth development when the impaction problem is noted. Surgical intervention is limited to those teeth still in the process of developing root structure (eruption). These teeth will benefit from the removal of the physical factors preventing eruption.

In the majority of cases, the simple excision of the fibrotic tissue covering the tooth bud will be all that is needed. When the impaired eruption results in a marked change in the alignment or direction of growth, a surgical repositioning of the developing tooth is indicated. Stabilization of the tooth following its movement is usually limited to sutures in the soft tissue. The lack of crown structure above the gingival margin makes anything else difficult. Other forms of stabilization would tend to inhibit the eruptive potential of the tooth.

When one discovers the impaction after the formation of the tooth root, the tooth has lost its power of eruption. Surgical procedures would be limited to the simple exposure of the crown to allow access for orthodontic appliances.

MAXILLARY CANINE ORONASAL FISTULA

The massive opening between the oral and nasal cavities, which becomes so obvious at the time the canine tooth is removed, is the end result of long-term periodontal disease. The animal will frequently exhibit signs of nasal foreign-body discomfort (sneezing) for a year or more before enough bone is lost for the tooth to loosen or abscess out of the socket. The chronic impaction of food debris will sustain a marked inflammatory response in the adjacent nasal structures as well as the osteitis of the maxillary bone. These reactions should be allowed to subside before attemtping to surgically close the fistula. Two months is usually necessary for this adjustment.

The fistula is surgically closed with a mucoperiosteal flap. The epithelial margin is scraped or cut away around the diameter of the fistula. Slightly diverging incisions are made from both the rostral and caudal margins of the fistula. The cut extends down through the mucosa, muscular structures, and periosteum. It is extended toward the bridge of the nose until a flap of sufficient length to cover the fistula is obtained. The periosteum is elevated from the bone margin dorsally, producing a flap that is unattached on three sides. The periosteum is cut at the apex of the flap. This enables the free periosteum with its attached soft tissue to be moved over the fistula. Interrupted sutures are placed around the flap margins. Care should be exercised to completely close all points on the suture line, particularly the corners.

Sutures are removed in 10 days. Few complications are likely. Occasionally, a part of the suture line will not heal, and a small fistula will re-establish itself. If the area is only a few millimeters across, it may not warrant added surgery. If the area is large enough to make closure desirable, wait another 2 months before attemping to repeat the closure. Antibiotics are seldom needed.

SIMPLE TECHNIQUES FOR ORAL WIRING

With few exceptions, the fractures of the oral cavity can be handled effectively with wire techniques. A few basic conditions must be met for wiring techniques to achieve bone repair and restore oral health. When these are obtainable in an individual case, the more involved techniques of bone plates, intermedullary pins, acrylic plates, extra-oral devices, or total oral immobilization are not necessary. When these conditions cannot be fully met, other techniques should be considered.

First, the teeth must be returned to a functional position. Usually this would be the previous position of the teeth of the individual, although sometimes improvements can be realized. In all cases, the final position of the teeth must be such that no pressure is transmitted to the bone structure by the teeth closing into occlusal contact. When conditions will not allow stabilization in the original position, the change in dental relationship must be such that this rule is met even if it means loss of additional tooth or bone substance.

Second, the soft tissue of the oral cavity must protect the bone from the oral microorganisms. Of the physical conditions that fall under this category, perhaps the most frequently encountered is a soft-tissue defect that occurs at a fracture site. While the soft tissue will fill a defect over intact bone, the presence of wires, plates, and so on in a soft-tissue defect will lead to problems in a majority of cases. Mucosal tissue flaps, extraction of teeth, and reduction of the height of the alveolar bone are methods of gaining free tissue to cover the stabilizing materials. Another condition in this category is the fracture line that extends into or through an alveolar socket. The gingival tissue and periodontal ligament have a difficult time reattaching to the tooth root quickly enough to prevent seepage of oral fluids into the alveolus and exceeding the contamination the bone can withstand. This is particularly true when pre-existing periodontal disease has destroyed alveolar bone or when existing alveolar osteitis reduces the capability of the bone to repair. Again, extraction of teeth is necessary in fractures of this type. The tissue adhesives, which were recently introduced into veterinary supply lines, offer a method of increasing the closure and sealing procedures for oral tissues. Although they do not replace sutures for strength, they are much more effective in stopping oral contamination of fracture sites around teeth.

Third, one must stabilize the oral fractures. This can be achieved in two ways—by applying the materials to the teeth and letting the bone heal to the stable tooth roots or by applying the materials directly to the bone. Either way, stability is as important in oral fractures as in any other process of bone repair.

Fourth, one must avoid trauma to soft tissues and teeth in the repair attempts. Much has been written of the delicate nature of the periodontal tissues and their inability to completely recover from injuries. Fracture repair techniques that inflict injury on the periodontal tissues usually result in periodontal disease in the area within a few years or, if periodontal disease already exists in the mouth, an increased rate of tissue destruction. The same can be said of injury to the tooth structures themselves. The enamel and dentin of the crown can be manipulated without long-term physical effects, but the damage to the pulp tissues and dentin of the root is not tolerated well. Fracture repair materials should never be placed into or within these tissues.

MANDIBULAR SYMPHYSIS REPAIR

Fracture lines around and through the mandibular symphysis can be stabilized with the same technique. The mandibles are correctly positioned, and a figure-eight wire around the lower canines is tightened down lightly. This holds the lower jaws in correct position during the next steps. The animal is placed on its back, and the ventral surface of the chin is clipped and prepped for surgery. An incision about 1 to 1.5 inches long is made. By centering the incision over the posterior border of the mandibular symphysis, both mandibles can be accessed through the same incision. Moving the incision over one mandible, the periosteum is incised and reflected off the ventral surface of the mandible. A hole is drilled through the mandible, just below the ventral cortex and just posterior to the end of the symphysis. A no. 1 or 2 round bur is large enough to permit a 24- to 26-gauge wire to be passed through the mandible. The skin incision is rolled to the other mandible and the process repeated. The wire is passed through both mandibles, and the posterior ends of the symphysis are brought firmly together as the wire is tightened. The wiring of the posterior symphysis stops the up-and-down movement of the fracture as well as the anterior-posterior movement. The skin is closed over the wire ligation and the animal is returned to lateral or ventral recumbency. While checking the occlusal contacts, the figure-eight wire around the canines is tightened firmly. This will equalize the pressure along the symphysis and assure fracture stability. The intraoral wire is left in place for at least 3 weeks.

The essential points of success are to have the mandibles aligned and to properly position the posterior holes. If the holes are not equally placed just posterior to the end of the symphysis, tightening of the wire will move the incisors out of proper position. The holes must be just below the ventral cortex to avoid possible injury to the apical end of the roots of the lower canines. Complicating factors would include the cases in which the palate is also fractured and there is traumatic loss of the lower canine(s). When the canines are broken, they should be left in place until the symphysis heals before attempting extraction of root fragments. In fact, by inserting a post in the root canal, even a severely fractured canine can serve as support for the intraoral wire during repair of the symphysis. If the canine is absent, the incisors can be wired together to stabilize the anterior symphysis or bonded together with composite resin restorative material material during the healing phase.

MIDLINE PALATAL FRACTURES

Most of the simple, midline palatal fractures require no repair if the occlusion is correct. Although shifts in the dental relationship occur with a palatal fracture, a single circum-maxillary wire is often all that is needed to retain correct tooth position during bone healing. The circum-maxillary wire is placed just behind the canines for the cat and as far back in the premolar area as the anatomy will allow for the dog. Placement is achieved by inserting a long, slightly curved needle through the skin on the dorsum of the nose. The needle is pushed down to the periosteum and moved laterally along the periosteum until it passes off the top of the maxillary bone. It is passed along the lateral surface of the maxillary bone and down into the oral cavity. The needle should exit the soft tissue just above the mucogingival junction and between teeth. Take the needle off the oral end of the wire and replace it on the free end of the wire. Place the needle back through the same skin hole and walk it off the opposite side of the bridge of the nose, along the side of the maxilla and into the other side of the oral cavity. By bringing the end of the wire across the palate and tightening, equal compressive pressure is achieved around the whole maxillary structure.

When tightening the wire, care must be taken to ensure the correct tooth position. Too much pressure on the wire will cause the maxillary canines to tilt lingually, interfering with the lower canines as they close. Just enough pressure should be applied to bring the margins of the palatal fracture close together; more pressure forces the edges to overlap rather than to just meet. Palatal soft tissue can be sutured if it appears necessary, but usually it is not.

MANDIBULAR BODY FRACTURES

Most fractures of the body of the mandible occur as a single fracture line, usually on a slight angle either anterior-posterior or buccolingual, or both. In the absence of extensive periodontal disease, one or two wires across the fracture line will restore stability. Interdental wires can be added if needed or sometimes used in place of one or more cross-fragment wires. When more than one fracture line is present, the placement of multiple wires may be required. In general, the re-establishment of a stable top and bottom cortical plate line is the goal of wire placement.

Don't hesitate to remove teeth from the fracture area. Adherence to the basic principles is essential as the complexity of the fracture increases or as complicating factors, such as existing periodontal disease, are encountered. A fracture is occasionally encountered where the fracture involves the developing tooth bud of a permanent tooth as well as the deciduous tooth already in the dental arch. In general, if a permanent tooth bud has been grossly contaminated, partially dislodged from its base, or prevents the establishment of a stable fracture line, it should be removed. In no case should materials used for stabilization be placed through a developing bud or be placed in the path of eruption. It is better to remove the bud than to block its eruption or have it abscess from contamination or injury received during the fracture process.

MANDIBULAR ANGLE AND CORONOID PROCESS FRACTURES

All of these fractures should be handled with fragmental wiring techniques. No matter how complex these fractures are, the re-establishment of the dorsal/anterior and ventral/posterior cortical lines is required. The fracture lines involving the very thin area of the coronoid process can be ignored, particularly those above the level of the temporomandibular joint. The approach from the ventral midline of the mandible, with reflection of soft tissue both medially and laterally, will allow access to these fracture sites.

Fractures involving the articulating surfaces of the temporomandibular joint can be successfully handled by amputation of the mandibular condylar head. This area will form a false joint similar to the hip joint. Attempts at repair, although initially successful, often result in the long-term deposition of arthritic bone. With this comes temporomandibular joint pain, reduced oral opening and function, and eventual muscle atrophy. It is better to effect permanent relief with amputation than to face the chronic debilitating process of temporomandibular joint dysfunction.

EXTREME SITUATIONS

When cases occur that present extreme problems, such as bone fragmentation too small to wire or massive loss of soft tissue or bone, healing by second intention often provides the best chance for a successful outcome. The placement of a pharyngostomy tube for administering food and water along with the liberal use of antibiotics for 2 or 3 weeks will frequently allow the body to establish a functional state. Usually the mouth is left unsupported, although bandaging the muzzle, wiring the jaws together, or partial wiring of the fractures may be indicated.

Results often considered to be failures of healing can still leave the animal with adequate oral function to comfortably sustain life. In this category would be such things as a functional nonunion in the body of the mandible, removal of a mandible, and loss of substantial amounts of palatal/maxillary bone. The animals adapt to many situations initially appearing hopeless and do very well as pets.

ORAL APPROACH TO VENTRICULOCORDECTOMY

The removal of the majority of the vocal cords produces a dog with greatly reduced vocal volume and pitch. The noise that remains can vary from just a rush of air to about one third of the preoperative volume. The procedure is quick, easy, and usually permanent if done properly. The loss of vocal capability seems to have no effect on the personality or behavior of these animals and, in the urban environment, often means the difference between being able to exist as a pet or being rejected. Chronic barkers will continue to go through the motion of barking just as a declawed cat continues to exercise its forepaws on scratching posts.

Three factors determine the clinical ease of performing the surgery—anesthesia, light, and instrumentation. Any of several injectable anesthetics or gas anesthesia can be used. The depth must be adequate to block the cough reflex while entering and manipulating the trachea. An agent that reduces peripheral blood pressure seems to reduce hemorrhage to a nominal amount. The vocal folds are not easy to visualize with most surgical lights. A "head lamp" light source that can concentrate the light output in a narrow beam along the line of sight will provide the best illumination. The instrument of choice is a human cervical biopsy punch. The handles should be 11 to 14 inches long with the normal scissor-type ring grips. The biopsy basket should be about 4 by 7 mm. This will be adequate for 15- to 20-pound dogs and larger.

When adequate anesthesia has been achieved, the dog is placed in sternal recumbency. Tongue and head control is essential to easy access. Surgeons with large hands can hold the tongue with the thumb and three fingers, leaving the forefinger free to prop against the roof of the mouth. This will allow maximum tongue extension and give the ability to control head position with one hand. Smaller people may need to use a mouth speculum or have an assistant hold the mouth open. The biopsy forceps are positioned with the vocal fold between the jaws. The fold is removed by taking multiple bites with the forceps, starting about one fourth of the way off the ventral border and removing the top three fourths at the fold. The fold should be cut close to the posterior border, and particular attention should be paid to removal of the cartilaginous portion on the dorsal margin of the vocal fold. After the process is repeated on the opposite side, the dog is returned to lateral recumbency and the head allowed to hang over the edge of the table until the hemorrhage stops.

Several things make the technique easier to accomplish, including extreme extension of the tongue and maximum spread of the jaws. The nose is elevated and the occipital crest depressed until the trachea and the lower jaw are straight. Then, when the epiglottis is depressed with the forceps, the vocal folds are easily seen and accessed. The tongue is grasped with the palmar surface of the hand and fingers against the dorsal surface of the tongue and the thumb under the tongue. A gauze sponge is needed to ensure a good grip on the tongue. The forefinger supports the maxilla just behind the canine tooth. The biopsy forceps are held with the blades working in lateral directions and the palm of the hand under the handles.

Postoperatively, a few dogs will cough small blood clots infrequently for several hours and the clients should be cautioned to keep the dog in an area where blood spots will not cause a problem. Soft foods are suggested for 2 or 3 days, although most will go back to their normal diets immediately.

The only complications that may be seen are a gradual return of volume if the cords regrow or the animal learns to use other tissues to produce noise. If the vocal folds are cut too close to the floor of the trachea, a few will heal across the trachea. They will eventually build a thin, soft-tissue wall across one half to two thirds of the trachea. The tissue can be trimmed out with the biospy forceps, but regrowth is frequently seen. The only permanent solution for some of these animals is to surgically open the trachea from the ventral midline, trim out the offending tissue, and pull a mucosal flap across the cut surfaces to prevent the side-to-side healing of the area. Few dogs have any significant hemorrhage. Most stop within a few minutes and lose only a few drops. If hemorrhage becomes a problem, insert an endotracheal tube and position the cuff over the cut surface. Inflating the cuff applies pressure to the cut surface, and gas anesthesia can be continued until the bleeding is controlled.

Dogs may be debarked at any age. Dogs debarked early in life tend to have a greater incidence of regrowth of the vocal folds. Dogs that have the surgery after 4 or 5 years of age seem to hemorrhage a little more than the younger animals.

Veterinary Dental Clinic
9695 S.W. Freeway
Houston, Texas 77074

0195–5616/86 $0.00 + .20

Oral Surgery

Radical Resection of Maxillary and Mandibular Lesions

Colin E. Harvey, B.V.Sc., M.R.C.V.S. *

Until about 10 years ago, oral tumors were treated surgically by resecting the protuberant soft-tissue lesion, leaving the underlying bone intact. Because almost all oral tumors on gingival or palatine surfaces invade bone locally, conservative surgical treatment resulted in almost universal recurrence, even for benign lesions such as epulides. Because of these poor results, other treatment modalities came into fashion. It has taken several years of accumulation of case data for it to become obvious that nonsurgical treatment methods are rarely any more successful for malignant lesions than conservative surgery alone.

Some oral tumors (fibrosarcoma, epulides) invade bone locally but are slow to metastasize; if the limits of the lesion can be estimated accurately, these lesions are ideal candidates for aggressive local therapy. Other oral tumors, such as squamous cell carcinoma and particularly malignant melanoma, metastasize earlier, and local treatment, no matter how aggressive, must be combined with regional or systemic therapy to control metastases.

Probably because of concerns regarding disfigurement and inability of the animal to prehend and swallow food, development of techniques for the radical (en-bloc) surgical resection of maxillary and mandibular lesions in dogs and cats proceeded slowly until recently. Recent experience at the Veterinary Hospital of the University of Pennsylvania[2, 4] and other veterinary hospitals[1, 6–11] has shown that these techniques are practical and not particularly difficult

*Diplomate, American College of Veterinary Surgeons; Professor of Surgery, Department of Clinical Studies, University of Pennsylvania School of Veterinary Medicine, Philadelphia, Pennsylvania

technically. These techniques provide the opportunity for complete removal of a malignant lesion, including the zone of microscopic invasion that results in recurrence following less radical procedures. Dogs and cats are surprisingly tolerant of these procedures. The quality of life provided by these procedures is good to excellent.[1, 2, 4, 6-11] The multiple anesthetic episodes required for radiotherapy and the systemic sickness and multiple office visits required for chemotherapy are avoided.

Temporary occlusion of both carotid arteries through an incision in the neck should be considered if extensive surgery is likely,[5] particularly in an animal in poor condition or anemic because of blood loss from an ulcerated lesion.

Oral tissues have an abundant blood supply and an epithelial surface that is constantly bathed by saliva, a fluid rich in antimicrobial protection systems. Healing of incisional wounds in oral mucosa is more rapid than for skin. Infections following oral surgical procedures are very rare, even though the oral surfaces cannot be prepared prior to surgery with the same attention to detail available for skin preparation, and postoperative cleanliness by isolating the affected area is impractical.

The purpose of this article is to describe the techniques and complications of maxillectomy and mandibulectomy and to summarize results from several series of cases.

MAXILLECTOMY

The term "maxillectomy" is used here to refer to the removal of any part of the upper jaw that includes teeth. Bone actually resected can include part or all of the maxilla, incisive bone (premaxilla), palatine bone(s), and vomer. Part of the nasal septum is included in some maxillectomy procedures.

The procedure commences with an incision in the palatal, gingival, and buccal mucosa to outline the extent of resection, which should be at least 1 cm away from gross margins of the lesion (Fig. 1A). If the incision is located close to the zygomatic or parotid duct openings, the ducts are identified by placing a length of monofilament suture material into the duct lumen; the glands can be sacrificed by ligating the duct, if necessary, or the transected duct can be transferred to a new location. The epithelium is reflected to expose the underlying bone. Hemorrhage is often profuse, particularly when the palate is incised. The major palatine artery can be seen, clamped, and ligated once the palatine incised edges are reflected. Hemorrhage from other areas can be controlled by pressure until the resected tissue is lifted out, when the vessels themselves can be

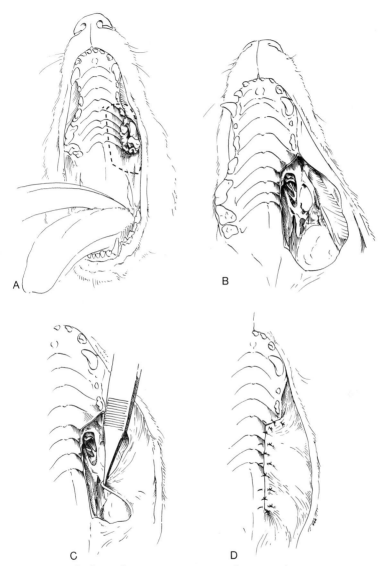

Figure 1. Radical maxillectomy. *A*, Lesion with proposed incisions. *B*, Extent of resection; the nasal cavity and orbital tissues are visible. *C*, Creation of the buccal flap. *D*, The flap has been sutured to cover the oronasal defect. (From Harvey, C. E. (ed.): Veterinary Dentistry. Philadelphia, W. B. Saunders Co., 1985; with permission.)

located and ligated or electrocoagulated. Electrocoagulation should not be used on the incisional edges that will be sutured later, for dehiscence is more likely.[7] The maxilla and palate are fractured along the incision lines with a diamond wheel in a dental handpiece, an osteotome, or an oscillating bone saw (Fig. 1B). The line of incision may include the infraorbital canal. If so, the infraorbital artery is identified and ligated. The tissue to be resected is levered up, remaining attachments are separated, and the section, usually including several teeth in situ, is removed en-bloc.

The nasal passage normally will be exposed at this point if the resection is adequate. Resection that does not expose the nasal cavity is unlikely to be adequate as primary treatment of a maxillary oral malignancy. Hemorrhage is controlled, blood clots are removed, and the remaining tissues are examined. If there are areas of turbinate that were partially severed or traumatized during the resection, they are cut with scissors to leave a clean edge. Hemorrhage that cannot be controlled by ligation or pressure may respond to surface application of 5 per cent cocaine solution. Use of dilute epinephrine is not necessary and is to be avoided, particularly when the anesthetic agent used is halothane.

The defect between the nose and mouth is covered with a buccal flap that is created by incising the buccal mucosa and undermining it until sufficient tissue is formed to cover the defect without tension (Fig. 1C). Most of the connective tissue layer is left attached to the buccal mucosa to ensure viability of the flap in its new position. My personal choice for apposing the tissues is a combination of vertical mattress and simple interrupted synthetic absorbable sutures (Fig. 1D). Other suture patterns have been used, with little evidence that the pattern itself was of importance; disruption was found to be more common when the incision was made with an electroscalpel.[7] Drains are not necessary. The connective tissue surface of the flap that faces the nasal cavity heals by granulation and epithelialization of the nasal mucosa.[7]

Radical maxillectomy may result in a loss of most of the lateral external skeleton of the nose, and the soft-tissue flap closed across the defect may cause obstruction of nasal airflow. If this appears likely at the time that the flap is created, sections of nasal conchae can be resected with scissors to create free air space in the reformed nasal cavity. The bone forming the conchae is very delicate; tissue that is to be retained should not be retracted or crushed by sponges.

This procedure can be adapted for lesions penetrating into the orbit by extending the resection to include the entire infraorbital canal and adjacent bone, infraorbital fat, and zygomatic salivary gland.[3] Closure is as described in the preceding section.

Following bilateral radical premaxillectomy, the defect between the oral and nasal cavities can be covered by creating unilateral or bilateral buccal mucosal advancement or rotation flaps. If bilateral flaps are used, the flaps are placed so that both cover the oronasal defect when sutured together, one with the epithelial surface facing dorsally to form the floor of the nasal vestibule and the other with the epithelium facing ventrally to form the new palate surface.[10] This double-flap technique is more involved than single-flap closure and has not been found to be necessary.[2, 6] As for maxillectomy, part of the ventral nasal conchae may need to be resected to retain space for air movement in the nasal cavity following closure.

POSTOPERATIVE CARE AND COMPLICATIONS

The animal may be in pain during the recovery from anesthesia but is usually able to eat without difficulty the following day. Breakdown of the sutures holding the flap in place may occur 2 to 4 days following surgery. If wound disruption does occur, the animal is reanesthetized and the flap is resutured. If an oronasal fistula persists, it does not necessarily result in dysphagia, as some animals adapt well when fed particular types of food.[2] If there are persistent problems with nasal regurgitation, another attempt can be made to cover the defect by creating a new flap from a different area once the original incisional edges have healed. Feeding the animal through a pharyngostomy or gastrostomy tube is of doubtful value in preventing dehiscence. Antibiotic administration is not necessary. The animal should be fed a soft diet and prevented from chewing hard objects for several weeks following surgery to protect the flap while it heals.

LONG-TERM RESULTS

Of the 60 animals included in three case series summarized in Table 1,[2, 6, 11] none were euthanatized because of inability to eat or drink or disfigurement. Eleven of 60 dehisced, most commonly when the surgical site was located caudal to the second premolar tooth. Because the lip on that side is pulled more medially than normal, the canine tooth may ulcerate the lip mucosa. If this bothers the animal, the tooth can be shortened or extracted.

The major complication is recurrence of disease. None of the animals with benign disease reported to date have developed recurrence (see Table 1). For the animals with malignant lesions, long-term survival was greatest in animals with squamous cell carcinoma (7 of 11 were alive or dead of other causes an average of 14 months

Table 1. *Results Following Maxillectomy in Dogs and Cats*

LESION	NUMBER	MEAN SURVIVAL TIME (MONTHS)	RESULT
Malignant Lesions			
Malignant melanoma	5	9 (range 1–20)	4 e/d dis
			1 a/doc
Squamous cell carcinoma	11	11 (1–28)	4 e/d dis
			7 a/doc
Fibrosarcoma, neurofibrosarcoma	18	9 (1–31)	13 e/d dis
			5 a/doc
Osteosarcoma	5	13 (4–28)	3 e/d dis
			2 a/doc
Undifferentiated sarcoma, carcinoma,			1 e/d dis
anaplastic sarcoma	4	11 (1–27)	3 a/doc
Benign Lesions			
Epulis, odontogenic tumors,			
adamantinoma, ameloblastoma	11	16 (7–34)	11 a/doc
Osteoma, osteomyelitis	2	16 (14, 19)	2 a/doc

Data from references 2, 6, and 11.
e/d dis = euthanatized or died due to recurrence or metastasis.
a/doc = alive or died of causes not related to oral lesion.

following surgery); recurrence was common in animals with malignant melanoma and fibrosarcoma, although even in those dogs and cats, the survival times were longer than those reported following other treatment methods, and included 6 of 18 animals with fibrosarcoma that lived longer than a year following surgery. Several of the animals included in Table 1 were treated with radio- or chemotherapy in addition to maxillary surgery.

MANDIBULECTOMY

Provided that an appropriate diet is given, the mandible is not essential for survival in pet dogs or cats. If a significant portion of the rostral end of the mandible on both sides is lost, the tongue hangs forward, and the animal (dogs in particular) may become a very messy eater, may drool frequently or continuously, and may not be able to groom itself normally. Similar effects are seen following removal of a large mandibular segment on one side in dogs, as the tongue loses its lateral support. This latter effect can be counteracted to some extent by shortening the commissure of the lip,[10] as described in the following section.

For lesions located in the premolar or molar area, hemimandibulectomy is performed.[1, 4, 10] By removing the entire mandibular bone on that side, the possibility of recurrence due to extension of tumor into and along the medullary cavity is avoided. In cats, hemimandibulectomy is easy to perform. The larger vertical ramus in dogs makes it easier to perform horizontal ramus segmental mandibulectomy in this species, although total hemimandibulectomy should be used if there is any likelihood of invasion of the medullary cavity. For either technique, incisions are made well away from the lesional tissue in the free gingiva (Fig. 2A), and the mandible is undermined by blunt dissection. The symphysis is separated by bone cutters or scissors (Fig. 2B), and the lateral attachments of the tongue are separated, leaving the mandibular and sublingual gland ducts intact if they can be identified. This frees the mandible so that it can be swung independently, which facilitates dissection of the masseter and pterygoid muscles from their attachments (Fig. 2C). These muscles are reflected laterally and medially, respectively, exposing the vertical ramus of the mandible.

For horizontal ramus segmental mandibulectomy, the mandible is transected caudal to the last molar tooth, and the mandibular alveolar artery in the medullary cavity is located, clamped, and ligated. For total hemimandibulectomy, exposed or incised vessels, including the mandibular alveolar artery, are ligated and dissection of the mandibular attachments is continued. The temporomandibular joint ligaments are exposed by rotating the mandible (Fig. 2D) and transected so that the mandible can be removed from the surgical site. A drain can be placed in the cavity beneath the suture line, exiting through the skin. The incision is closed by absorbable sutures apposing the incised oral mucosal edges (Fig. 2E).

To retain lateral support for the tongue in dogs, the mucocutaneous junction of the lip on that side is incised both dorsally and ventrally as far forward as the first or second premolar teeth, and the incision is extended into the connective tissue to form flaps. The mucosal flap of the dorsal lip is sutured to the mucosal flap of the ventral lip with absorbable sutures, and the skin flap of the dorsal lip is sutured to the skin flap of the ventral flap. The closure can be buttressed by placing absorbable sutures in the connective tissues before commencing placement of the skin sutures. Tension-relieving devices such as button sutures have been suggested as a means of avoiding dehiscence.[10]

For benign or very localized malignant lesions located in the incisor or canine tooth area, a rostral mandibulectomy is performed. The buccal mucosa is incised to allow the mandible to be undermined, the mandible is transected with an osteotome or diamond dental wheel caudal to the first premolar tooth to avoid the curved root of the canine tooth, the mandibular alveolar artery within the medullary cavity is ligated, the sublingual mucosa and lingual muscles are incised (avoiding the mandibular and sublingual salivary ducts if possible), and the mandibular segment is removed. Bleeding

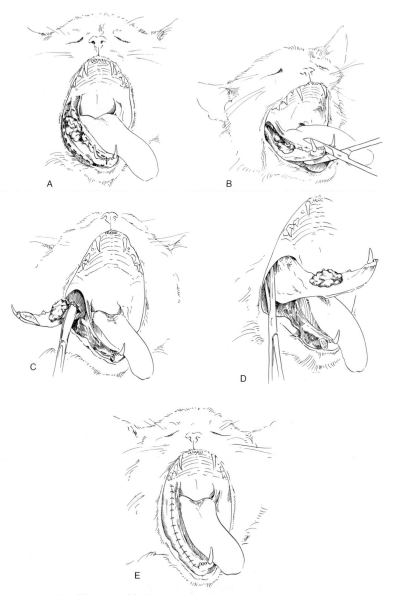

Figure 2. Total hemimandibulectomy in a cat. *A*, Lesion and proposed incisions in the mucosa (*dashed lines*). *B*, The mandibular symphysis is split. *C*, The mandible is rotated to facilitate muscle dissection. *D*, The lateral ligament and condylar attachments are separated. *E*, The mucosal incisions are sutured. (From Harvey, C. E. (ed.): Veterinary Dentistry. Philadelphia, W. B. Saunders Co., 1985; with permission.)

vessels are coagulated or ligated, avoiding the use of electrocoagulation on the mucosal edges that will be sutured. The buccal and sublingual mucosal incised edges are sutured with absorbable sutures. The cut surface of the mandible should be covered completely by soft tissue if possible, which may require placement of sutures around teeth to hold mucosal flaps in place.

Rostral mandibulectomy can be performed unilaterally or bilaterally. The use of orthopedic appliances such as screws, pins, or wires to maintain stability of the remaining mandibular segments is not necessary[4, 10] and may result in pin or wire migration later.

Following resection of mandibular segments, the remaining mandible will drift medially, but dogs and cats accommodate readily to this. If the remaining mandibular canine tooth impinges on the palate when the mouth is closed, 2 to 3 mm of the crown can be filed down without exposing the pulp cavity, or the tooth can be extracted. A soft food diet probably will be necessary for the duration of the animal's life, although the animal is able to eat and swallow by itself.

The coronoid process of the vertical ramus of the mandible can be resected without disturbing the horizontal ramus.[3] The incision is made over the zygomatic arch, the periosteum of the arch is elevated, and the arch is resected using a bone saw, diamond wheel, or rongeur. The temporal and pterygoid muscles lying rostrolateral and medial to the coronoid process are reflected. The coronoid process is transected as needed, and the incision is closed by suturing the zygomatic arch periosteum to the orbital fascia.

RESULTS AND COMPLICATIONS

Table 2 summarizes the results of mandibulectomies in 71 dogs and cats treated in five veterinary hospitals.[1, 4, 8–10] One cat undergoing hemimandibulectomy died as a result of hemorrhage during the procedure itself. Two cats and one dog were unable to eat or drink satisfactorily and died or were euthanatized; all of the other 90 animals were able to prehend and swallow satisfactorily. Dehiscence of the lip commissure narrowing incision occurred in one dog. Drooling and grooming abnormalities were present in some animals but were not severe enough to result in euthanasia. Prosthetic replacement surgery was performed 6 months following horizontal hemi-mandibulectomy in one dog.[9]

The long-term results depended on the pathology present. All 23 animals with benign disease were alive or had died of unrelated causes at follow-up (mean 28 months). For the malignant lesions,

Table 2. *Results Following Mandibulectomy in the Dog and Cat*

LESION	NUMBER	MEAN SURVIVAL TIME (MONTHS)	RESULT
Malignant Lesions			
Malignant melanoma	20	9 (range 1–44)	11 e/d dis 9 a/doc
Squamous cell carcinoma	30	14 (1–54)	9 e/d dis 21 a/doc
Fibrosarcoma, neurofibrosarcoma, spindle cell sarcoma	14	14 (1–50)	8 e/d dis 6 a/doc
Osteosarcoma, chondrosarcoma	11	10 (1–30)	11 e/d dis 2 a/doc
Lymphoreticular tumor, mast cell sarcoma, histiocytoma	5	13 (5–38)	3 e/d dis 2 a/doc
Benign Lesions			
Epulis, ameloblastoma, adamantinoma, myoblastoma	19	27 (11–66)	19 a/doc
Cysts and other benign disease	4	28 (12–60)	4 a/doc

Data from references 1, 4, 8, and 10.
e/d dis = euthanatized or died because of oral disease.
a/doc = alive or had died of other causes.

results were best in animals with squamous cell carcinoma (21 of 30 were alive or had died of other causes; mean follow-up 18 months).

SUMMARY

The results obtained following both maxillectomy and mandibulectomy in animals with benign disease show that these procedures are practical. The challenge is to select those animals with malignant disease where the disease is sufficiently localized so that radical resection will be curative, or where residual disease can be controlled by adjuvant therapy. The series of cases reported in Tables 1 and 2 represent animals treated during the "developmental phase" of these procedures. With 5 years of case experience now available, the usefulness and limitations of these procedures are becoming clearer.

REFERENCES

1. Bradley, R. L., MacEwan, G., and Loar, A.: Mandibular resection for removal of oral tumors in 30 dogs and 6 cats. J. Am. Vet. Med. Assoc., *184*:460–463, 1984.
2. Emms, S. G., and Harvey, C. E.: Preliminary clinical experience with maxillectomy in dogs and cats. J. Small Anim. Pract., 27:291–306, 1986.
3. Harvey, C. E.: Veterinary Dentistry. Philadelphia, W. B. Saunders Co., 1985.
4. Penwick, R.: Clinical experience with mandibular resections in dogs and cats. Submitted to J. Am. Vet. Med. Assoc., 1985.

5. Hedlund, C. S., Tangner, C. H., Elkins, A. D., et al.: Temporary bilateral carotid artery occlusion during surgical exploration of the nasal cavity of the dog. Vet. Surg., 12:83–85, 1983.
6. Salisbury, S. K., Richardson, D. C., and Lantz, G. C.: Partial maxillectomy and premaxillectomy in the treatment of oral neoplasia in the dog and cat. Vet. Surg., 15:16–26, 1986.
7. Salisbury, S. K., Thacker, H. L., and Richardson, D. C.: Partial maxillectomy in the dog: Comparison of suture materials and closure techniques. Vet. Surg., 14:265–276, 1985.
8. Vernon, F. F., and Helphrey, M.: Rostral mandibulectomy: Three case reports in dogs. Vet. Surg., 12:26–29, 1983.
9. White, R. A. S., Gorman, N. T., Watkins, S. B., et al.: The surgical treatment of bone-involved oral tumors in the dog. J. Small Anim. Pract., 26:693–708, 1985.
10. Withrow, S. J., and Holmberg, D. L.: Mandibulectomy in the treatment of oral cancer. J. Am. Anim. Hosp. Assoc., 19:273–286, 1983.
11. Withrow, S. J., Nelson, A. W., Manley, P. A., et al.: Premaxillectomy in the dog. J. Am. Anim. Hosp. Assoc., 21:49–55, 1985.

Department of Clinical Studies
School of Veterinary Medicine
University of Pennsylvania
3800 Spruce Street
Philadelphia, Pennsylvania 19104

0195–5616/86 $0.00 + .20

Establishing a Veterinary Dental Practice

Gary Beard, D.V.M.*

The most common questions asked of those who have developed a veterinary dental specialty practice are "How do I get started?" and "What kind of equipment should I buy and where can I buy it?" These are very simple questions on the surface, and with most specialities, simple answers are involved. Not so in veterinary dentistry. In veterinary school, we learned the basics, such as anatomy and physiology, but we lacked instruction on the application and skills needed in clinical practice. All too often, it boiled down to "If the teeth are dirty, clean them, and if they are loose, pull them." No consideration was given to the basic tenets we find in all other specialties—mainly, "How can I improve the health and well-being of the patient by application of my skills and knowledge?" We were taught to go to almost any lengths to save the functions of an eye or a limb or any other part of the anatomy except the teeth.

Dentistry is one of the oldest specialties known to human medicine, yet we in veterinary medicine have virtually ignored the benefits and, consequently, the devastating effects of poor oral health on the entire body system. We can no longer ignore oral health and hygiene when attending to the total health and well-being of the patients in our care.

Prior to 1977, when the American Veterinary Dental Society was formed, there was little interest in dentistry and even less information on what to do, how to do it, and where to obtain the materials necessary to implement the needed procedures. We had to borrow techniques and equipment from our colleagues in human dentistry. There was even less information on the veterinary applications of this specialty. To date, we have made significant progress.

---

*Goodwood Animal Hospital, Baton Rouge, Louisiana

There are numerous seminars given monthly that are spearheaded by the American Veterinary Dental Society, the American Animal Hospital Association, Eastern States, Western States, and even the Animal Medical Center in New York. Equipment and material needs are being adequately met by a number of dental supply companies. The Henry Schein Company has led in the development of equipment and materials; they have even developed "kits" for various procedures and publish a veterinary dental supply catalog.

GETTING STARTED

There is an old Louisiana saying that pertains to cooking Cajun specialties: "First, you make a roux." Essentially, it means that you develop the basics first and build from that solid foundation. We have the basic veterinary knowledge in anatomy, histology, and physiology, and we only need to develop the skills and art needed for the specialty. It has already been mentioned that there are numerous programs available in almost all regions of the country introducing the interested practitioner to what is possible and practical to do. We are fortunate that the clients and patients are already in place. All we really need to do is to build from the basis of human dentistry and extrapolate the client education that has gone on for years to our own use. We are constantly reminded as consumers of dental services that oral health is necessary both for our total body health and for aesthetic reasons. Over 100,000 dentists and the national news media constantly remind us of what we need to do; they also remind us that saving teeth is more healthful than extracting teeth.

Dr. John McCarthy, past-president of the American Animal Hospital Association, included veterinary dentistry in his President's Message of February, 1984:

If only one half of our present clientele found the need for only one additional visit to our hospitals each year, we would be overwhelmed with work. To do that, we only need to convince our clients of the real need for dental prophylaxis, recognizing problems before they become major, or the benefits of good preventive care.

According to Mark Tholen, D.D.S., in his book, *Concepts of Veterinary Dentistry*, "85 per cent of all animals over six years of age have periodontal disease. By treating these animals, the practice gross can be increased 10–15 per cent without adding any new clients."

Dr. Tom Mulligan, in a paper presented at the 52nd Annual Meeting of the American Animal Hospital Association in Orlando, Florida, reported that in a 17-month period following his special interest in dentistry, his practice income from dentistry increased over 390 per cent. His return on investment of money spent on dental equipment and supplies was 831 per cent. Therefore, the initial step in the process of how to get started is already in place: the clients are there waiting for you to further educate them about total health care for their pet.

In the American Animal Hospital Association manual of standards, the basic tenets state that "dental services will be provided," and most of us do provide basic services such as dental prophylaxis. The proper manner in which to conduct a dental prophylaxis is pointed out in other sections of this issue. We need to supplement this with the most important ingredient of "making our roux"— client education. The first time a puppy or kitten is brought in for a visit, we should start educating our clients on the dental needs of the patient: deciduous teeth that hopefully will be completely extruded, the need for home dental hygiene, the importance of diet, the early recognition of problems that can arise, and what to do in case of traumatic injury. It is our place to point these things out and remind clients that dental care similar to what they receive is necessary and available to their pets.

Next, your new clients and clients with mature pets should be included in your program at each visit. A thorough examination of the oral cavity should be a part of every visit regardless of the reason for that visit. To state that the oral health is good and a dental prophylaxis is not necessary at this time goes a long way toward establishing the basis for a procedure when the need arises.

There are three good veterinary dental textbooks available at the present time.[1, 2, 3] A thorough knowledge of the contents of these books is a necessary adjunct to the initiation of a special interest practice.

One of the most important first steps is the recording of dental data. Outlines for numbering and nomenclature are given in the dental texts.[1, 2, 3] A word to the wise is in order here: keep it simple, but be accurate. Proper dental terminology and nomenclature are absolutely necessary to communicate effectively with dentists and other veterinarians with whom you might consult. After developing a dental record and acquiring knowledge of dental terminology and anatomic relationships, you should become intimately familiar with normals. Whether you are dealing with ophthalmology, cardiology, or dentistry, you must first know and recognize normals. You should become acquainted with the structure, dentition, and position in different species; you should also recognize differences in breeds. Abnormalities will be obvious once you master the normals.

It will be advantageous to next categorize the various areas of interest you will want to develop and the depth or level at which you want to operate. Just as in other specialties, you must define the point at which, in the best interest of the client and patient, you refer the case to a veterinary dental consultant. For simplicity, you can break down the areas of interest into these four classifications:

1. Periodontics, which includes routine dental prophylaxis; client-conducted oral hygiene and home care; more involved procedures such as subgingival curettage and root planing; gingivectomy; and radiographic procedures.

2. Endodontics and restoratives, which include root canals; caries; pulp capping (for fractures and disarming); fracture repair; root amputation; and re-implantation.

3. Orthodontics and dental orthopedics, which include interceptive orthodontics (selective extraction); malocclusions (congenital versus hereditary); dental impressions and models; types of appliances; bonding and adhesives; and mandibulectomy.

4. Oral pathology, which includes neoplasms; stomatitis and other soft-tissue lesions of bacterial or viral origin; and gingival hyperplasia.

I offer, at this point, a pearl of wisdom that will help you immensely in bringing your specialty practice to fruition: Establish and maintain a good relationship with your dental colleagues and their paraprofessional personnel. The dental hygienist is an invaluable aid in the training of your technicians in the proper way to conduct a prophylaxis, including root planing, curettage, use of the ultrasonic scalers, and care of dental instruments. Continuing education of this sort is invaluable and has the advantage of being done at your own practice without expensive travel. Don't hesitate to show your appreciation by offering to pay for this service and, in all ways, retain this good relationship.

The question of what kind of equipment to buy and where to buy it is easier to answer today than it was a short time ago. In fact, we are faced with so many alternatives now that we are limited only by what we want to accomplish and how much we want to spend.

I mentioned earlier in this article Dr. Tom Mulligan's approach, in which he outfitted his office with full dental services and equipment. His success after careful preparation was phenomenal. Other practitioners have approached veterinary dentistry in a more gradual manner and have been equally successful, but over a longer period of time. I believe that, for most veterinary practitioners, the gradual approach of mastering certain techniques and associated instruments and material is the best course to follow. Just as with other aspects of veterinary medicine, there are numbers of ways to accomplish an end. Know your basics and try to improve your technique. This applies to instrumentation as well (you can accomplish good, if not a better, dental prophylaxis with hand scaling instrumentation than with an ultrasonic scaler). In fact, you and your personnel should become thoroughly familiar with hand instrumentation before you purchase an ultrasonic scaler, which should only be an adjunct to treatment.

In preparing for endodontic therapy, you must decide what type of power source you will use for drilling into the tooth for access to the pulp cavity. This same equipment can be used for polishing teeth after a prophylaxis, cutting teeth, cutting and shaping appliances, and many more uses, but it can be very expensive.

Most dentists use air-driven equipment, which requires an air source, such as a compressor. It can generate speeds up to 400,000 rpm and is very versatile with low- and high-speed handpieces available. The disadvantages are that it is costly and an area is needed to house the compressor. For those of us who have reached a level of skill that requires speed and state of the art equipment, this may be the best equipment to purchase.

For the practitioner developing a special interest in veterinary dentistry, the electric-drive units serve well in every way. The cost is very reasonable and they are self-contained, mobile, and can be sterilized and used for certain orthopedic procedures.

Once you have resolved the major purchases of the ultrasonic scaler and the unit for drilling and polishing, the other selections, while more numerous, are certainly less expensive. Few procedures that you will be doing in veterinary dentistry involve more than a few cents to a few dollars in material. The only notable exceptions are the caps, bridges, and appliances that you may have to purchase from a dental laboratory. I can think of no specialty that has a greater potential for profit from procedures performed than dentistry. You should base your charges on time cost per procedure, just as the human dentist does.

To list all of the equipment and supplies needed for your dental practice would take too much space and would be redundant in light of the excellent catalogs available from Henry Schein, Inc., and other suppliers.

To simplify your choices and minimize your initial financial outlay, kits are available that will allow you to perform most of the procedures that you will deal with on a daily basis in your practice (Figs. 1 to 11).

For instance, Henry Schein, Inc. offers a Veterinary Oral Surgery Kit (Fig. 3), Veterinary Periodontal and Endodontal Kit (Fig. 7), and a Dental Care Unit, (Fig. 1) (electric-drive drilling and polishing unit) for under a thousand dollars. These kits can be supplemented with other instrumentation as you improve and expand your procedural abilities. A Veterinary Ultrasonic Scaler (Fig. 2) will

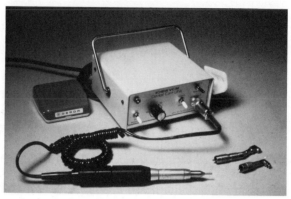

Figure 1. Schein VC-30 Dental Care Unit, which is used for obtaining access into the pulp cavity, polishing the teeth after prophylaxis, driving numerous drills, cutting and grinding burs and wheels.

cost approximately $595.00 (Schein) (Fig. 2). The Cavitron 2002 will cost approximately $875.00.

Other items involved in specific procedures (endodontics, orthodontics, and so on) will be discussed in other articles in this issue.

At the end of this article is a list of a number of dental supply houses that handle equipment and/or materials for dental use. There are also suppliers in most locales from whom you can obtain new and used equipment. Your dental consultant will be an excellent source for this information.

One area that I feel is very important and should be mastered early on in your dental specialty is that of making impressions and models. Dental models are an absolute necessity for making appliances for orthodontic procedures and are excellent for use in con-

Text continued on page 1004

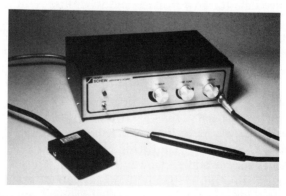

Figure 2. Veterinary ultrasonic scaler. It accepts all cavitron-style inserts. It is used for scaling teeth and, with attached TEN-10 Tip, for removal of subgingival calculus.

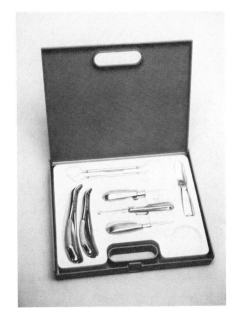

Figure 3. Veterinary oral surgery kit. The kit includes extraction forceps, periosteal elevator, tooth elevators, bone curette, root tip pick, and tissue retractor.

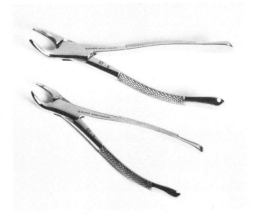

Figure 4. Extraction forceps.

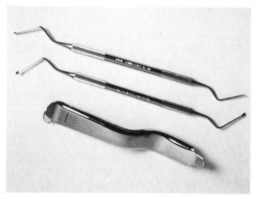

Figure 5. Bone curette, root tip pick, and tissue retractor.

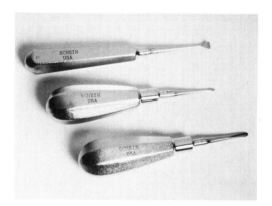

Figure 6. Periosteal elevator, small tooth elevator, and large tooth elevator.

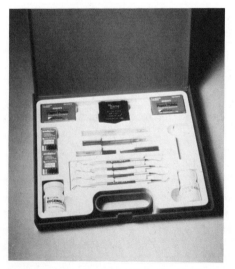

Figure 7. Veterinary periodontal and endodontic kit. It includes dental hoe, scalers, explorer/probe, zinc oxide, eugenol, paper points (short and long), 25-mm files, irrigation needles, filler needles, and mylar composite tape.

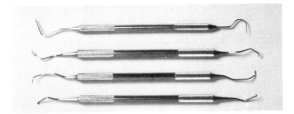

Figure 8. Explorer/probe, scalers, and dental hoe.

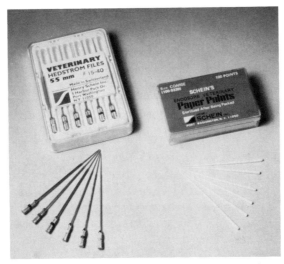

Figure 9. 55-mm files and long paper points. They are necessary for root canal therapy of canine teeth.

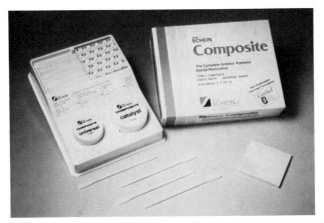

Figure 10. Composite restorative, which is used for filling cavities, restoring enamel erosions and hypoplasia, and rebuilding fractured teeth.

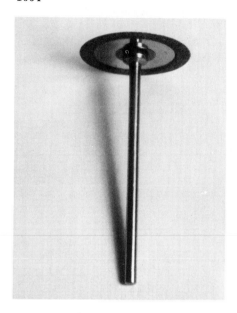

Figure 11. Cutting disk on mandrel. It is diamond-coated to easily section multirooted teeth and is used with VC-30 Dental Care Unit.

sultation and referrals. For years, some of us have sent models to practitioners who had more expertise than we had. With these models and a verbal and written description, consultative advice is available. In addition, you may have a dental laboratory make appliances that are not available in your practice area.

The following are basic materials needed for impressions and models:

1. Impression trays: Human trays can be used if they are built-up or deepened by adding dental wax to the rim; or Form-a-Tray (various suppliers) custom tray for various-sized animals.

2. Mixing bowls: Flexible rubber or plastic (various suppliers).

3. Spatula: Metal blade with a smooth, rounded end to reach every part of the bowl curvature, and a wooden or plastic handle.

4. Dental materials: Dental wax for preparation of rim of impression tray (soft utility wax); alginate (normal or medium setting speed); dental stone material (pink is stronger); gypsum hardening liquid (makes stone harder than when using water).

5. Plastic knife: Must be sharp for trimming models.

6. Vibrator: For even filling of impression to avoid bubbles and faulty models.

Impressions are an exact replica of the animal's mouth and must be done under anesthesia. Again, read and become familiar with the procedures, then have your dental consultant or his technician go through it with you. If impressions cannot be filled with stone immediately, they should be kept moist until they are poured.

Once you have mastered the techniques and skills required and the pertinent questions about the basics of "setting up a dental practice" have been answered, the next question to ask is "How do I inform my colleagues and potential clients of my services?"

First, I believe you should inform your colleagues, who are potentially your best source of referrals. A personal letter to each practice in your area specifying that you have a "special interest" in dentistry and would appreciate consultations and referrals on dental cases would be appropriate. Volunteering to deliver a program on veterinary dentistry to your local association would further enhance your position plus a position protocol on your handling of cases. Don't forget that clients will travel long distances for services not available in their own area, so do not neglect to inform regional colleagues as well as local. After you have fully informed the veterinary community, you may wish to talk to various kennel and feline fancier clubs, as well as breed-associated clubs. Just as in other areas of specialties, word-of-mouth referral from satisfied clients will become your largest single source of referrals.

Make every effort to ensure that your clients are fully informed of what can and cannot be accomplished and have reasonable estimates as to costs involved and time estimates in more involved procedures such as capping, restorations, and orthodontics.

Always remember that dental surgery is surgery, and appropriate laboratory tests and consent forms are necessary as in other surgical procedures. Establish a good working relationship with a human dentist and his dental technician. Most are more than willing to share their expertise with you and your personnel. Most of all, be willing to learn new techniques and continue your education for your practice lifetime. This is a sure-fire guarantee to prevent burn-out and ensure a profitable and enjoyable practice of your veterinary dental special interest.

SOURCES OF DENTAL MATERIALS

1. Dental supply houses (new and used equipment) in all large cities.

2. Mail order: Henry Schein, Inc.
5 Harbor Park Drive
Port Washington, New York 11050

Hot line for Veterinary Dental Supplies
1-800-872-4346

Servet, Inc.
P.O. Box 246
South River, New Jersey 08802
(201) 257-8505

Harry J. Bosworth Co.
53 South Plymouth Court
Chicago, Illinois 60605

Arista Surgical Supply Co., Inc.
67 Lexington Avenue
New York, New York 10010
(212) 679-3694

Deepen Enterprises, Inc.
Veterinary Dental Supplier
P.O. Box 389
San Mateo, California 94401

Pulpdent Corporation of America
75 Boylston Street
Brookline, Massachusetts 02147

Lincoln Dental Supply Co.
1319 W. Nedro Avenue
Philadelphia, Pennsylvania 19141
(215) 549-7470

Jeremy Ethan Industries, Inc.
P.O. Box 956
Woodside, New York 11377
(718) 886-4367

DVM Doggy Dent
111 St. Matthews Ave.
San Mateo, California 94401
(415) 342-2976

Alrich-Girard Corp.
24634 Fire Mile Rd.
Redford, Michigan 48239
(313) 533-8253

3. Endodontic materials:
> Union Branch Dental Products
> 3640 37th Street
> Long Island, New York 11101

4. Orthodontic materials:
> Rocky Mountain Dental Products
> P.O. Box 1887
> Denver, Colorado 80201
>
> Unitek Corporation
> 2724 South Peck Road
> Monrovia, California 91016
> (213) 445-7960
>
> Codesco, Inc.
> 1234 Market Street
> Philadelphia, Pennsylvania 19107

5. Dental engines:
> Foredom Electric Co.
> Bethel, Connecricut 06801
> (203) 748-3521

6. American Veterinary Dental Society
3850 Spruce St.
Philadelphia, Pennsylvania 19104
Colin E. Harvey, B.V.Sc., M.R.C.V.S., Secretary

REFERENCES

1. Eisenmenger, E., and Zetner, K.: Veterinary Dentistry. Philadelphia, Lea & Febiger, 1985.
2. Harvey, C. E. (ed.): Veterinary Dentistry. Philadelphia, W.B. Saunders, Co., 1985.
3. Tholen, M. A.: Concepts in Veterinary Dentistry. Edwardsville, Kansas, Veterinary Medicine Publishing Co., 1983.

Goodwood Animal Hospital
8778 Goodwood Boulevard
Baton Rouge, Louisiana 70806

Index

Note: Page numbers of articles and issue title are in **boldface type**.

Changing Your Address?

Make sure your subscription changes too! When you notify us of your new address, you can help make our job easier by including an exact copy of your Clinics label number with your old address (see illustration below). This number identifies you to our computer system and will speed the processing of your address change. Please be sure this label number accompanies your old address and your corrected address—you can send an old Clinics label with your number on it or just copy it exactly and send it to the address listed below.

We appreciate your help in our attempt to give you continuous coverage. Thank you.

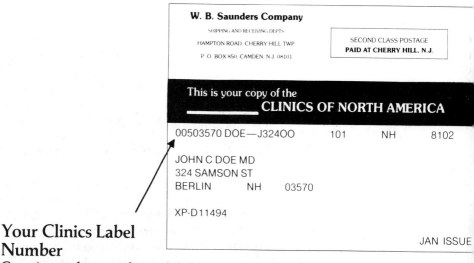

W. B. Saunders Company

SHIPPING AND RECEIVING DEPTS

HAMPTON ROAD. CHERRY HILL. TWP

P. O. BOX 850. CAMDEN. N.J. 08101

SECOND CLASS POSTAGE
PAID AT CHERRY HILL, N.J.

This is your copy of the

_____ CLINICS OF NORTH AMERICA

00503570 DOE—J32400   101   NH   8102

JOHN C DOE MD
324 SAMSON ST
BERLIN   NH   03570

XP-D11494

JAN ISSUE

Your Clinics Label Number

Copy it exactly or send your label
along with your address to:
W. B. Saunders Company, Fulfillment Services
West Washington Square, Philadelphia, PA 19105.

Please allow four to six weeks for delivery of new subscriptions and for processing address changes.